A PRACTICAL GUIDE TO BREATHWORK

A REMEDY FOR THE MODERN HUMAN CONDITION

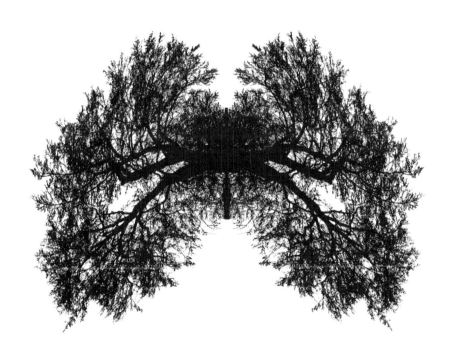

JESSE COOMER

FOREWORD BY KASPER VAN DER MEULEN

Contents

Foreword

Every. Single. Breath...

Determines the level of metabolism in your mitochondria.

Influences the pH level of your blood and tissues.

Communicates through the brainstem to every thought and emotion you feel.

Is electrically wired through the heart to influence every beat.

Exchanges vital information between your environment and your immune system.

Informs your nervous system on which organ functions to activate or suppress.

Determines the quality of your thoughts, attention and actions.

Massages each organ in your abdominal cavity through movement of the diaphragm.

Literally pulses your brain and spinal fluid up and down.

Influences your blood pressure and level of vascular dilation / constriction.

Regulates the levels of inflammation in the body.

Is an opportunity to come back to your center.

Is a tool to express yourself authentically.

Sets the pace for how much calm or anxiety you experience.

But mostly: Every single breath - and with it, all of the above - could be under your conscious control. And we live in an exciting time to do so.

For thousands of years many scholars, yogis and spiritual teachers have known about these amazing ways that each breath influences our human experience. However, this information was not always readily available to the public. Even in modern times breathwork was often vailed in vague terms, clouded by rituals or simply kept away from students until they were advanced enough.

When I personally was caught by the power of the breath about 6 years ago, it improved my life in every possible way, and I felt it was time to spread the word. The first thing I realised was that breath was like a missing link in the health, fitness and performance world. I thought to myself *"how is almost everybody missing this?!"*

Even some of my clients who were at the pinnacle of human performance, like special operations and Olympic athletes, were overlooking the power of breath. They optimised their training, nutrition, sleep, supplementation and mindset. But when it came to breathing - literally the most important thing you do - they were so underdeveloped that I could easily help them "hack" their performance in a few sessions. Not because I'm such a genius coach, but because it was the lowest hanging fruit for them.

Since my first encounters with breathwork there has been a massive upsurge in the interest for and openness to this field of work. It is no longer considered vague, woo or new-agey to work on your breathing. The ever-growing scientific interest into respiration has created a modern, tangible and clear understanding that supports and explains many of the benefits that the ancients knew of, in a language that us westerners can get behind.

At the same time, a paradigm shift is slowly happening. In the self-development and human optimisation world, there was always a massive focus on the mind: positive thinking, goal setting, visualisation, affirmations, self-talk, mindfulness etc. have been the main topics of focus. And - though they are undeniably powerful tools - they often disregard physiology.

Through practicing and studying the breath, you will soon learn that the mind is a function of the brain, and the brain is part of the nervous system. And your nervous system determines the state of your physiology, and your physiology largely determines how well your mind functions. Through the unique human function of consciously changing the way you breathe, you gain access to the deeper laying functions of the "automatic pilot" that is your physiology. So, I'm not saying that there's anything wrong with these "mind" techniques, I'm saying that they become far more powerful when you start to use them from the breath.

But then which technique is the ultimate technique? Which method should you focus on? How do you find your path in the seemingly endless forest of different protocols?

Thanks to the growing scientific understanding of breathing, and the diligent work of excellent researchers and teachers, it is becoming clear that these may not be the right questions. Slowly but surely the world of breath is evolving to an amazing new place. A place where the boundaries between techniques, brands, opinions and methodologies are fading away. Fading away to make place for a greater understanding, a larger picture: a paradigm of principles.

You see, every single breathing protocol is built on the same foundation of very clear and simple core principles. Once you understand these principles and pair them up with practice, you will develop a keen understanding of which techniques are right for you, and when you should use them.

So nowadays you are no longer dependent on finding the right teacher who holds the big secret truth, you don't have to humbly serve the guru to get the real techniques and you certainly need not sit in a cave for 30 years to figure it out for yourself. The remote control to your nervous system, the operating system of your mind, the regulating dial of your human experience is right there within you, within every single breath.

All you need is a curious mind, a willingness to practice and a book just like this one to get started.

In this book Jesse Coomer has skillfully brought together those core principles, and some of the most powerful techniques that you can dive straight into. As you read these pages and the valuable information within them, remember that every single breath brings with it the potential to change your life. Every. Single. Breath.

Kasper van der Meulen

The Breathwork Biohacker

www.KaspervanderMeulen.com

Introduction:
How to Read this Book

"What a piece of work is man, How noble in reason, how infinite in faculty, In form and moving how express and admirable, In action how like an Angel, In apprehension how like a god, The beauty of the world, The paragon of animals." - Prince Hamlet to Rosencrantz and Guildenstern

Congratulations on Your Inheritance!

Welcome, my fellow human. Much has changed since our ancestors first stood upright and walked the Earth. You are the descendant of the countless humans who came before you, all of them with their stories, their aspirations, their dreams, and their troubles. And your Neolithic Grandparents have left you a gift, an inheritance passed down through the ages through the language of DNA.

The fact that you are alive today is one part of your inheritance. In short, we hail from a long line of people who were at least somewhat proficient at not dying. Just think about that for a minute. There is an unbroken chain of mothers and fathers that stretch from the very first human being to you. This unbroken chain came with a great deal of struggle and difficulty, and here you are, the beneficiary.

You have also inherited a body and mind that have been tested in every environment that this world has to offer, equipped with onboard mechanisms that were evolved to suit the world humans first found themselves in. Your fellow humans have lived in desserts, rainforests, remote archipelagos, frigid tundra, and moderate four-seasoned climates that change dramatically throughout the year. Equipped with complex internal systems and a sturdy physical frame, your ancestors not only survived life on this planet, they thrived amid a world of uncertainty, filled with fierce predators and food scarcity.

So, now here we are, endowed with a body and mind that is perfectly suited for life on Earth. A precious gift that took thousands of generations to arrive here, today, for you! But we no longer live in the same world for which this gift was designed. The modern world is a completely different place to live.

So, did we get a bad inheritance? Like an old VCR? Of course not. We just need to be able to understand how to adapt this gift so that it works well with the environment in which we now live.

The purpose of this book is to explain some of the conflicts that arise between our evolutionary programming and modern life and why conscious breathing, also known as "breathwork," is such an effective tool for the modern human.

The Modern Human Condition

The "human condition" is a term used to describe all of the essential events, emotions, and feelings of the human experience. Our fears, our hopes, our passions, they unite us as a species because we can all relate to experiencing these aspects of being human. The human condition knows no border, and it reaches across the ages. We can pick up a translation of Sumerian Epic of Gilgamesh written in 1,800 BC and relate to the friendship described between Gilgamesh and Enkidu. Love, friendship, envy, greed, these are all things that we feel and have always felt. These universal attributes of the human experience affect every aspect of our lives.

For those of us living in modernized societies, I submit that we have a new shared experience, something I call "the modern human condition." The disconnection between a hunter/gatherer species and the modern world is something we all share, but we have only recently begun to detect it. We have built incredible societies, developed medicines, and have even sent some of our species to the moon, but the more we seem to thrive as a species, the more we seem to suffer in other areas of life, as a result. The "modern human condition" is that we are living in an environment of our creation to which our species has yet to adapt, one that seems to solve all of the problems of survival but has unwittingly created other dangers. In this book, I detail some of the most common disconnections between our modern world and our ancient human programming. It is this disconnection that we share with all humans living within modern societies that I call the "modern human condition".

How to Read this Book

This book is broken into two halves. The first half is focused on the modern human condition, how it affects our lives, and why breathwork is such an incredible tool to reduce the negative effects of the modern human condition and live a better life.

The second half of this book (starting with Chapter 12) is a practical guide to breathwork. **You don't have to wait until you are done reading the first half in order to begin your breathwork practice.** While reading the first half will help you gain a deeper understanding of the mechanisms at play in your breathwork practice, I wanted to make the breathing techniques and protocols available to you as soon as you pick up this book. If you want to read the first half in concert with reading the second half, by all means, do it! My purpose in writing this book is to add as much value to your life as possible through this medium.

Breathwork is your birth right. We are born with incredible capabilities, but we are never given an operator's manual. May this book serve as an operator's manual for how you can use your breathing to improve your life. This isn't a textbook filled with an information overload. There are already lots of books like that. This book provides you with the information that you really need to understand the modern human condition and to use breathwork to live a healthier and happier life. It is the book I wish I had when I started my own breathwork journey. May every breath you take while reading it bring you happiness.

Chapter 1.

No Rest for the Worried

A bed is a wonderful thing, an invention that has been perfected over the centuries. It is probably the most important piece of furniture that we will ever buy. In commercials and magazine ads we see happy people, eyes closed, sleeping blissfully on the latest reinvention of the mattress. A light blue hue of moonlight peeks through the draped window as the happy sleeper… demonstrates how to use a mattress.

Do we really need a demonstration of this? Perhaps there are some people out there who see the ad and wonder, "how am I supposed to use this device?" However, for the rest of us, the sleepers in the mattress commercials are selling us on a promise: if you buy this mattress you will sleep as peacefully as the people in the picture seem to be sleeping. Yes, the paid actors in the advertisements are there to sell you on the idea that the quality of your sleep depends on the comfort of your mattress.

Of course, they're not wrong. There is a reason why we buy mattresses. If you've ever had to sleep on a really hard or uncomfortable surface, you know that it can be enough to keep you up all night. Even though every mattress store I have ever seen seems to be throwing a "going out of business sale," mattresses are not a fad. Humans like sleeping on comfortable surfaces.

So why are we constantly tossing and turning in these comfortable beds of ours? Why are so many sleeping drugs out on the market? What drives us to taking valerian and melatonin every night? If being physically comfortable were the secret to sleep, why are so many of us still missing out?

While there are many causes for a poor night's sleep (all the parents with newborns know of at least one cute and utterly helpless one), the most common reason that people share with me is that they can't get their minds to "turn off." I think all of us can relate.

It's as if our minds are waiting for our heads to touch our pillows, and then suddenly all of the problems in life that didn't seem so out of control before we closed our eyes must now be solved as we try to go to sleep. We think about how we will address a problem at work tomorrow or which words to use in an email that we have to write. Somehow our minds won't let us sleep tonight because tomorrow needs to be figured out right now.

Or maybe you're like me, and you think of something stupid you said or did five years ago. Or maybe it was twenty years ago. Why am I thinking about this right now? Those people probably don't even remember that it happened… or maybe they do. Maybe they have been judging me ever since, and I'm just a fool who does stupid things. And everyone knows!

Other times, we conjure up arguments that never happened; arguments that may never happen! We think of a person who holds a belief or a point of view that just drives us crazy. So instead of drifting into a blissful sleep like the people in the mattress commercials, we host a CNN style debate in our minds. We think of the perfect way to "mic drop" our opponent. And just when we believe we have won the imaginary debate, we think of something else we could have added. Or we remember another thing about the person that we can't tolerate. And round two begins!

And the whole time, we might be lying on the most comfortable mattress that money can buy. Teams of mattress engineers probably worked tirelessly on your mattress, creating perfect support for your lumbar and thoracic spine, balancing softness with firmness, and knitting a perfect top to ensure that your body remains cool throughout the night. And there you are, telling Connie from the office that her political view isn't as well thought-out as her smug face thinks it is.

It's all enough to make me wonder if those people in the mattress commercials are really sleeping blissfully either. Maybe they are just like the rest of us, trying to get to sleep despite the best efforts of their mind that just won't leave them alone.

Eventually, somehow, we fall asleep. And then suddenly the alarm clock wakes us up, and we begin our day, poorly rested. But that is okay because we can drink coffee, full of everyone's favorite drug, caffeine. And caffeine is awesome! It wakes us up, helps us poop, and makes us forget all about our habitually poor sleep for just one more day.

Value of Self-examination

People love quoting Socrates, who once said that "an unexamined life is not worth living." I admit it, I love spitting out this quote too, especially in my day job as a professor of English.

My job is to instruct college freshmen and sophomores in college level writing at Vincennes University, a small university in southern Indiana. The classes I teach are nothing fancy. Just some survey of literature classes and the basic rules of grammar and essay construction. The very rules that I am habitually breaking in this book for dramatic effect. For instance, the previous two sentences were technically incomplete.

I give this advice to college students to get them started in the process of self-creation. In a world full of facsimiles, I try to encourage people to become individuals, which is easy to say, but really hard to do. It takes a lot of courage. It also takes a lot of work and self-examination, just as Socrates prescribes.

Rumination

However, self-examination has its dark side too. It is really easy to over-examine ourselves, our actions, our choices, and even our feelings. We get obsessed with self-examination. Did I marry the right person? Did I make a mistake getting my degree in finance? Was it wise to buy a house when I could have rented? Did I do the right thing? Did I say the wrong thing?

And just like that, self-examination, the same activity that helps us figure ourselves out well enough to make our own choices, leads us to a state of rumination. Rather than using self-examination to guide our actions, we become paralyzed in an infinite feedback loop of examination. What is more, in the cases I mentioned in the paragraph above, all of the questions are backwards focused, looking at choices we have already made. Looking back in time at our past choices puts us in the ultimate disadvantage because there is no way that we can make a choice in the past. Those choices have already been made, so this kind of examination often involves asking ourselves questions for which there are no obvious or clear answers.

So, what do we do? Do we simply let go of our troublesome thoughts, adopting a sense of peace that there are some things in life we can't know? For most of us, the answer is 'no'. We double down on our rumination, letting it become a regular part of our thoughts throughout the day, led by an irrational sense that if we just keep thinking about it, an answer will become clear.

But it never becomes clear, and it never seems to end. Rumination puts us in a state of anxiety that colors our interactions with others, with the world, and with our perceptions of ourselves. It makes us reactionary, fearful, and paranoid. It can make us guarded and defensive, and this can cause us to do and say things that we will regret later. And then we will probably just ruminate on those things too.

It is reasonable to conclude that we ruminate on the past in order to make better decisions in the future. This makes sense. We all know the value of reviewing our past decisions to learn from them. This is how we learn. If we made a decision that led to a positive result, it stands to reason that more actions like those will benefit us in the future. And if we made a choice that led to disaster, of course, we will want to avoid ever making that choice again. So, when we ruminate on past events, we can justify the practice to ourselves. We do it because we want to make better decisions in the future.

And speaking of the future, what is going to happen tomorrow? How will you respond to future problems or events? Will you have enough time to get your work done? What if you don't? What if you get your work done, but it is full of errors? How will you write that email tomorrow? Well, look at the time! It looks like it's time to head to bed to get some sleep. Good thing you have a new comfortable bed to sleep on. Rest your weary head and just wait until tomorrow to solve your problems, both real and conjured. Just lie down like the people in the mattress commercial. Close your eyes and smile as you drift off to a peaceful night's sleep.

Chapter 2.
The Dopamine Feedback Loop

Whether you sleep well or not, chances are that you, like me, have bouts of rumination. And it could be that you, like me, have lived most of your life dealing with a brain that "just won't shut off."

For me, rumination didn't stop with endless thoughts about my own actions. I ruminated on other people's actions too. Why did she use THAT emoji at the end of her text message? What does he really think about me? Am I being taken advantage of by my significant other? He is smiling at me, but is it a fake smile?

And at the end of all of this over-analysis, I'm left with the most intimidating question of all. What will I do? This question leads again to an infinite number of paralyzing answers. Which is the right one? Which one will lead to the positive result that I crave, and more importantly, which one will keep me from making the mistake that I fear?

Aesop tells the story of The Fox and the Cat. It's an ancient story that expresses the dilemma of over-analysis, which humans have faced for all of history due to our developed brains. One day, the Fox and the Cat are discussing their tactics for escaping the hunting dogs that occasionally come looking for them in their woods. The very intelligent Fox says that he can think of many different ways to get away from dogs, so many that he cannot even count them all.

The Cat, on the other hand, can only think of one way to escape. For a moment, the Fox feels proud of his superior intellect, with the ability to think of a variety of ways to escape, while the poor Cat is simply not as smart. Suddenly, they hear the howls of approaching hunting dogs. The Cat uses the only escape that he knows; he climbs up the closest tree and hides. But the Fox, with a head full of possible escapes, is left pondering which one is the best. Of course, some of the escapes might even be bad ones that would lead to an untimely demise at the hands of the hunter and his dogs. The Fox simply cannot decide which way to escape, even though his mind is full of many ideas. But which idea will work? Which idea won't work? Rather than take the chance of making the wrong choice, the Fox takes no action, frantically thinking through the long list of possibilities. Soon, the Fox is surrounded by the hounds and is left with no path of escape at all.

The Fox in Aesop's fable is caught in what we now commonly refer to as "analysis paralysis," the human tendency to analyze a situation so much that our analysis blocks any action. No, it isn't just you who cannot "turn off your brain." This is a problem that all humans have faced since the beginning.

And it isn't for no reason. This drive to analyze problems is written into the very wiring of our brains. Our impulse towards rumination is caused by dopamine, the very neurochemical that drives us to explore the world and solve problems.

I used to think dopamine was a reward chemical produced by our brains; something to signify that one's actions have led to a desired result. We have all heard about the "dopamine hit" we get from checking our phones every five minutes. That instant high leads to addictive behavior, and we find ourselves turning to social media to feel good.

This is not the case at all. Dopamine isn't about rewards. It's about motivation.

Within the motivation center of our brains, dopamine drives two primary behaviors: accomplishing goals and eliminating uncertainty. Of course, eliminating uncertainty is a very worthwhile goal. Just think of all of the uncertainty that our ancestors faced throughout human history. After all, uncertainty could mean danger. If we don't know what is in the bushes, how can we be sure that there are no lions hiding there? Dopamine is the little nudge that we need to get up and check to make sure the area is safe before lying down and going to sleep. It gives us the nudge that we need to stay focused on a goal, and reassurance that our actions are worthwhile.

But uncertainty isn't always about avoiding lions. Uncertainty could also mean discovering a new source of water just over that horizon, a compatible mate in the neighboring tribe, the fertile hunting grounds in the dark forest at the edge of the unknown. Yes, dopamine is always there to encourage us to make known what is unknown, to explore and to discover, and to continue taking actions that are aligned with our goals.

I'm sure you can see how dopamine affects us in the modern age. Instead of checking the bushes for bears, we are driven by an unrelenting force to double-check if we locked the front door or turned off the stove. Of course, don't forget to check your handful of social media apps as often as possible. We have to check the news every night to stay informed of what is going on in the world around us, because we cannot afford to be ignorant. We are compelled to eliminate uncertainty.

However, there is also value in uncertainty. Just because something is dangerous doesn't mean it isn't worth taking our chances. In fact, it is our dopamine that can cause us to take great risks, all in the name of exploring new places, meeting new people, or experiencing something desirable. We are driven by dopamine, not rewarded by it.

How does this relate to rumination? Well, sometimes the motivational system of the brain identifies an instance of uncertainty that is impossible to understand, or a goal that is impossible to achieve (like correcting a mistake in the past, knowing whether you made the "right decision," or knowing if you will have a positive outcome). And as luck would have it, the more uncertainty that we identify, the more dopamine our motivational system pumps out into our brains, filling us with an impulse to do something about it, even though we can't. And even though we intellectually might understand that there is no way to solve this given problem, our motivational system begins to identify this uncertainty as being even bigger than we thought it was! So, the motivational system releases even more dopamine to motivate us to solve this riddle or problem. But again, it cannot be solved, so... more dopamine, more rumination, still no way to resolve the uncertainty... you get where this is going. It is a feedback loop. It is in these times that we suffer the wrath of the same system that is designed to encourage us to reach our goals.

Gambling is one of mankind's oldest ways to take advantage of the dopamine feedback loop, and bookies and casinos have made millions off of this wiring within our brain's circuitry. While writing this book, I was fortunate enough to meet Dr. Otto Muzik, professor of neurology in the School of Medicine at Wayne State University. He used the example of gambling to illustrate how the dopamine feedback loop drives our thinking and behavior.

"Since the games are designed to be unpredictable," said Dr. Muzik, "your motivational network drives you to keep rolling the dice or pulling the lever forever, in the false hope that in the near future you will obtain enough information about the system so you can reliably predict when you will win or lose (meaning that now you will be able to predict a future outcome, which is the highest goal in human evolution). Thus, your brain's motivational network will continue to supply your brain with dopamine to keep playing. If you win, you feel satisfaction and want to take advantage of your new insight, only to be crushed by the loss in the next round. So, you try again to get to the bottom of things." This is the danger of the dopamine feedback loop. Even if we intellectually know that we can never reliably predict the future, our motivational network continues to give us encouragement to keep trying.

"Interestingly," Dr. Muzik went on to say, "this motivational network is also connected to your reptilian brain (specifically to specific homeostatic centers in your brainstem) that in situations of uncertainty releases the neurotransmitter norepinephrine which diffuses throughout the whole brain. When systemically released, norepinephrine causes all your brain networks to react with greater responsivity, making your brain more sensitive to the slightest perceptions with the intention to increase your ability to solve an uncertain situation. Unfortunately, this increase in overall sensitivity to stimuli is psychologically experienced as anxiety."

In the same way that the gambling addict is futilely driven to solve the uncertainty in gambling, we are driven to ruminate. Humanity has had to struggle with the fact that life is full of uncertainty. Human beings, like the Fox in Aesop's fable, are intellectually gifted with brains that can fathom infinite ways to approach this uncertainty. Thanks to our technologically connected world, we have even greater access to information, which means more uncertainty than we were probably designed to face. Our brains chemically drive us to continually seek it out, but, as we now know, this motivation pattern doesn't necessarily bring us relief. It burdens us with anxiety, paralysis, and endless rumination. Thanks, brain. I know you are trying to help, but you're driving me crazy.

The Danish philosopher Soren Kierkegaard once said that "anxiety is the dizziness of freedom." He understood the mechanism that causes anxiety well before we could describe it biochemically. Here we are, in a world of uncertainty, around other humans who are unpredictable, and with whom we wish to make friends, do business, and fall in love. It's no wonder we can't sleep at night. There is no mattress comfortable enough to cancel out a brain that has been reinforced by thousands of years of natural selection. We are anxious balls of dopamine and norepinephrine, addicted to life's uncertainties. How do we ever cope with such a plight?

The question now is: What do we do with this information? Do we sit and ruminate? Do we find ways to use this motivation system, while learning methods to mitigate the negative effects of the dopamine feedback loop? Many of us choose not to engage at all. This is where I found myself for most of my life. My strategy for dealing with my motivational network's dopamine hits was to disengage; to solve the problem of uncertainty by avoiding it.

Chapter 3.

My Disconnected Life |
The Modern Human Condition

People who knew me before my early and mid-thirties would describe me as care-free (even though I was bound by anxiety and self-doubt at every corner). They would not describe me as fit or active, and they would likely not describe me as healthy. Any muscle I had on my body was simply there out of anatomical necessity. Like, just to move from one couch to the next. I literally moved from chairs to cars to other chairs or sofas.

I am an extrovert. I like being with people, and I feel my best when I am with other people, as long as I'm not making a fool out of myself or being disliked. This has not changed. In my youth, I was the same way, but my brain wasn't done growing. I was awkwardly learning how socializing works, and I was really great at pointing out my own mistakes. In other words, my mattress was not enough to get me to sleep at night. I ruminated all the time, I dreaded going to high school, and I felt like every social interaction could go south at any moment. And all the while, having a strong social connection with people was what I wanted most. When I started drinking and smoking weed, a lot of that internal chatter quieted down, and I was able to be myself.

I didn't really see a downside. I had finally found a "bed" of sorts that was comfortable enough to "turn off my brain." I felt that I had finally found a way to escape discomfort, both physical and psychological. No longer was I uncertain about how the day would make me feel. I had found a way to control the outcome.

After a few years of this, I got high once... for about ten years. Yes, that is my joke about my addiction to an opioid prescription pain killer. It isn't a great joke, but I hope you didn't buy this book for the jokes. Yes, I was an addict for ten years of my life, and for much of that time, I felt that I had once again figured out how to make life comfortable and avoid ruminating thoughts. I had started seeing my mind as an enemy, something that needed to be suppressed. And for a while, it worked. But it didn't work forever.

It was during this time I realized that there was really no way to completely run from discomfort, physical or psychological. No matter how many pills I took, my pain, discomfort, heartache, and anxiety caught right back up with me. It wasn't because of the usual things we associate with drug and alcohol addiction. I wasn't in and out of jail. I wasn't in and out of rehab. I never stole money from my family. Actually, most of my family didn't even know I had a full-on addiction. People who knew me during my first 30 years of life might not even believe me when I say that I was a hopeless pill addict for ten years. I didn't have the usual outward signs.

One sign that I did have was a general lack of direction in life, and a lack of motivation. Of course, this makes sense. I was taking copious amounts of pills every day to quiet that part of my brain. The same motivational system that had been giving me anxiety was also the one I needed to work towards goals and explore possibilities. While I did finish college and I did always have a job, I might argue that this behavior was motivated more by my wanting to maintain my addiction than anything else. I had to protect this addiction or I would have to face not only the terror that was my discomfort and anxiety, but a new unknown: life without drugs. I had been on drugs for so long, what would happen if I stopped taking them? This was an uncertainty that I would solve the same way I solved the rest of life's uncertainties. I would avoid it.

At some point, I realized that it wasn't my anxiety and discomfort that created overwhelm. It was my quest to avoid them. Uncertainty wasn't becoming stronger; I was becoming weaker. My ability to adapt and endure during instances of stress, anxiety, or pain were atrophied to a degree that, even in my opioid-induced numbness, I was no match.

The only reason I share this piece of my life with you is to provide context. As I came out of addiction, I had no foundation of tolerance for anxiety. No tolerance for pain. My lifestyle of avoiding discomfort landed me in adulthood with the tenderness of a freshly healed wound.

The Modern Human Condition

I was really surprised when I learned that my destructive lifestyle wasn't actually counter to my biology. It was a reasonable result of my ancient neurological wiring colliding with our modern world.

We might not all become drug addicts, but I learned that we are all driven by this ancient wiring, which when combined with the modern world, often leads us into bad habits, unhealthy relationships, poor health, destructive lifestyles, and, of course, sleepless nights. This ancient wiring served our ancestors well. The proof is that we are all here. Our species survived. But our overwhelming success has come with a cost, the modern human condition.

My first step in learning to live in the modern world was to quit my addiction. I'm not going to go into great detail here, because this book is not concerned with getting off of drugs. The reason I tell you this is to let you know that I had to learn to handle life's anxieties from ground zero; I had to unlearn my dysfunctional way of living while inventing a new and healthy path.

My first real lesson in starting this path was that I had to face life's stressors head-on. I couldn't wait for them to come to me anymore. I met new people, and I began to discover why facing stress, rather than running from it, can be the best way to beat it.

Chapter 4.

Primal Human, Modern World

I couldn't believe my friend. Was he even a friend? Why did I call him a friend? But there he was, looking at me like what he just said to my face was a reasonable request. Like it was something friends do when they want to spend time together. Even to this day, I remember just how repugnant it sounded.

"Hey, man," he said. "Let's go to the gym and workout."

I just stood there making a confused face. We hadn't been friends for very long, and I wasn't sure we would have much of a future after that kind of talk. Why would anyone want to go to the gym and workout, first of all, and why would people do such a chore as a social act? What else did he want to do for fun, lawn work? Unclogging toilets? Exercise? Really?

I looked at him, and I had to ask, "Is going to the gym and working out something that you find to be fun?" As for me, I stayed clear of the gym. For me, exercise felt like punishment.

My attitude towards exercise started when I was a middle schooler, and I would play basketball for my school team. What did the coach make you do if you messed up? He would make you run. Or he would make you do push-ups and run. Or he would devise some other incredibly uncomfortable punishment, but they all had one thing in common. They all involved exercise. Exercise was the thing you had to do when you were messing up. The kids who didn't mess up didn't have to exercise. So, therefore, as far as I was concerned, exercise was punishment.

And let's not forget about how uncomfortable exercise is. First you have to exert way more energy than you want. Then you get out of breath and sweat. And if you sweat, you stink. And no one likes the stinky kid. It really just made more sense not to exercise at all. That way I could stay nice and comfortable and clean.

My belief that exercise was punishment started when I was in middle school, but it really started to hit me in high school. I went to a small Catholic high school, and I tried to play every sport they had, except for golf and soccer.

Soccer was a strange new game for Midwesterners in the 1990's. I didn't know how it was played, so I didn't play it because it would require learning, which I also found uncomfortable. I also didn't want to play it because it involved sprinting for long distances. Basically, it required two things I didn't want to do: learn and exercise.

I played baseball, basketball, track, and cross country, and by my junior year of high school, I quit all of them to go be in a rock band. I liked being in a rock band. There is no exercising in a rock band. And when you are in a rock band, you can drink and do drugs all the time! Which feels great! I was so glad that I had abandoned exercise and sports, and I decided then and there that I was just fine without them.

All of this ran through my mind as I waited to figure out what was wrong with this friend of mine. Had he never been to basketball practice? How could someone see working out—the purposeful act of being uncomfortable—as anything other than a chore? As punishment?

But I decided to go to the gym with him. This was mostly because, at this time in my life, I didn't have any other friends. He was my roommate, and while this "working out" idea seemed a little odd, he seemed like an otherwise decent human being.

I had a problem, however. I didn't have anything to wear to the gym. My life was so devoid of exercise that I literally only had street shoes; no gym shorts, no gym bag, no gym shirt. I had to borrow clothes and shoes just to go to the gym that day.

I made the joke that I would walk in his shoes that day. You know, looking back, he was a pretty good guy to let me hang out with him at all.

I hated every exercise we did. I couldn't wait for the whole thing to be over with. When it was all done, I did feel really good, but I was pretty convinced that it was simply because the chore was done. The punishment that we, for some reason, willingly engaged in was complete. Exhausted, I didn't even have the decency to untie the double knot in his laces when I returned his shoes. He still reminds me of this transgression to this day.

The reality is that I, like you, need physical exercise to be a healthy and functional human being. This is not a new discovery. As early as 400 BC, Hippocrates, the author of the Hippocratic oath that every physician must take, published his longest work, *Regimen*, where he states:

> Eating alone will not keep a man well; he must also take exercise. For food and exercise, while possessing opposite qualities, yet work together to produce health. For it is the nature of exercise to use up material, but of food and drink to make

good deficiencies. And it is necessary, as it appears, to discern the power of various exercises, both natural exercises and artificial, to know which of them tends to increase flesh and which to lessen it; and not only this, but also to proportion exercise to bulk of food, to the constitution of the patient, to the age of the individual, to the season of the year, to the changes in the winds, to the situation of the region in which the patient resides, and to the constitution of the year.

Even as early as 400BC, Hippocrates was on to me. I wasn't eating well. I wasn't exercising. And I wasn't feeling well. But, I didn't understand the connection between exercise, something that was very uncomfortable for me, and feeling good. What is more, I didn't understand the connection between living the modern sedentary lifestyle and feeling bad.

Hippocrates was observing another one of nature's little miracles, the body's ability to become stronger when stress is applied to it in the appropriate dose. This is known as the process of hormesis. We see the result of hormesis when muscles grow stronger and larger after regular weight training exercises, as bones become stronger and denser as a result of jumping, running, and heavy lifting. In reality, the initial stressor is damaging to the body. Muscles experience small tears that cause inflammation, which we experience as soreness. Our bones experience micro abrasions that we don't even notice, but over time, those of us who are active and who regularly stress our bodies through physical activity, will experience the body's amazing capacity to become stronger as the result of these tiny injuries. In the 21st century, there is a common misconception that "stress = bad," but in reality, there are some forms of stress that, if experienced in the right dose, can result in positive outcomes.

This kind of stress is commonly referred to as "eustress." However, the absence of these positive stressors also causes us to atrophy; we become weaker and less resilient when we lack these stressors. This is why exercise is so important to the modern human's wellbeing. When we challenge the body, we become healthier and more resilient, even though our bodies might send signals of discomfort to our brains. And when we do not challenge the body, despite our momentary comfort, we will sadly reap the deleterious results. This blew my mind when I first learned about it. Not only is it amazing that our bodies are capable of becoming stronger as a result of damage they incur when used (which is the opposite of what happens to any man-made machine), they become weaker if not used regularly.

But the thing that didn't make sense to me was why a beneficial activity such as exercise caused so much discomfort, while sedentary activities, which ultimately led to weakness, seemed comfortable. I mean, shouldn't my brain reward me for doing something that is good for me? This was my first real taste of the disconnection between the world my body was evolved to live in versus the modern world.

The discomfort and pain that comes with physical activity is there for a reason. It is there to warn you that you are causing damage and to keep you from damaging yourself so much that you cannot recover. Literally, the "pain" that causes the "gain" is there to inform you that you are experiencing physiological stress. It lets you know when you are reaching your physiological limits, limits that if ignored will lead to serious injury. Yes, even though we can grow stronger when we push ourselves, there are limits. And if we push past those limits, we negatively stress our bodies into injury and weakness. The discomfort that comes with exercise is there to keep us from pushing too far. When I experienced this discomfort early on in my days of exercise, it seemed to scream at me to stop. I had atrophied so far that simply doing any physical exercise seemed like an injury inducing stress. Like so many other couch potatoes who decided to make a change in their health, I had to relearn how to interpret these internal signals. I was beginning to understand one of the disconnections between my physiology and the life afforded to me by the modern world.

For most of human history, the word "exercise" would not mean what it means to us. The idea that one should engage in more activity than one had to would also seem ridiculous to Neolithic man. But unlike modern humans, for men and women of most of human history, life was a constant physical struggle. Their reward for being physically active was survival. It was not until humanity began to farm sometime around 10,000 years ago that people were able to sit down long enough just to catch their breath. This drastically changed the course of human history, and the result has been art, music, cities, and every other thing that a human can do when his basic food and water needs are met. Early humans dealt with the uncertainty of finding food. Farming and domestication were their answers.

Cravings, the Foundations of Civilization

Fast forward to today, and in developed countries, we have a problem that our ancient ancestors might have found laughably implausible. We are dying fat and sedentary. We are capable of ingesting days' worth of calories within a single meal if we want to. It's called an "all you can eat buffet"—a title that seems to have become a challenge to Westerners. I, myself, have entered such establishments with the mind to "teach these buffet owners a lesson," "to get my money's worth." Of course, one only needs to look around the buffet line to see that this is a plan that has been devised by everyone else there.

Not only have we been insanely successful in producing enough calories to eat, we have learned to hack into our natural inclinations to seek out specific flavors, such as sweet or salty. It is not an accident. The craving for something sweet and something salty is written into our genetic code.

Our earliest ancestors lived in places where these flavors were very scarce. Their environments were dry and hot, and they lived on herbivorous diets which lacked ionic sodium. Scientists believe that the pleasant taste of salt is an adaptation that helped the earliest mammals, and therefore our ancestors, to be encouraged to ingest enough sodium for proper cellular health.

This common table seasoning had a huge hand in the development of our civilization. Natural sources of salt drew animals, which led to worn game paths, which humans followed to find animals. Humans turned the game paths into roads, and they settled down nearby. Much of our early history was driven by our craving for salt, which facilitates many biological functions such as maintaining blood fluids and sending nerve impulses. When people started to replace the sodium-rich meat from hunting with a diet of farmed wheat and grains, humans realized that they needed to supplement this lost sodium by salting their food.

Salt was a scarce commodity in the ancient and classical eras, which led to a large salt trade as human civilization grew. Its uses grew too. It became a way to preserve meat for later eating, and it was commonly used in ancient Roman medicine as an antiseptic. In fact, a portion of a Roman soldier's pay was comprised of salt, known as *solarium argentum,* which is where the English word "salary" comes from.

As a currency, salt was used to buy everything, from goods to even people. Which is perhaps where the phrase "any person worth his salt" came from. However, just like their ancestors before them, early empires had a problem. They still didn't have enough salt in their diets. Driven by a biological need, they created great salt mines, and as time progressed, humans have been able to add a saltshaker to every table in the world.

Sadly, we no longer live in a world where sodium is rare, and this proclivity for salty foods is now linked to high blood pressure and heart disease. According to the American Center for Disease Control, about 90% of Americans aged two and older ingest more daily sodium than is healthy. The 2020 daily recommended allowance for sodium (and we are talking the ceiling, not the minimum) is 2,300 mg of sodium, with an ideal maximum of no more than 1,500 mg. The CDC also reports that 90% of Americans aged two years and older ingest an average of 3,400 mg of sodium per day.

To put these numbers into perspective, in order to stay alive, the average human only needs between 150mg to 500mg of sodium. This, of course, will vary depending on how much a person is sweating, but the citizens of developed countries generally live in temperature controlled environments and do not engage in a high degree of physically demanding activity where perspiring this common electrolyte is a serious problem. So, lack of salt isn't a big killer in the modern world. Instead the modern human condition is to live in a world where salt is abundant while our biological drive for salt is still as active as ever, leading us to overconsume.

Sweetness is My Weakness

The urge for sweetness is also written into our genetic code. In its natural form, sugar is almost always attached to nutrition and energy in the form of fruit. In the earliest days of our human ancestry, it is believed that fruit was scarce in comparison to vegetables.

I love watching survival shows. It is amazing to see people improvise alongside nature in order to stay alive. I don't, however, think it would be fun to star in one. Sometimes, I watch episodes while eating my lunch. While the people in the show are starving and struggling to get by, there I sit, just munching away, enjoying the 30 to 60-minute program. I don't know why this seems like a fun way to spend a lunch break, and I promise I'm not a terrible person. I promise.

The one thing that is always a game changer on one of these shows is when they find fruit. The sugars in fruits and berries provide a much-needed energy boost for the poor saps, and they often even break into tears and smiles when they bite into the very elusive orange or berries.

Again, we have to put ourselves in the shoes of the people who came before us. If something tasted sweet, it was likely to be a great source of caloric energy, and not just any kind of calorie, either—easily-absorbed calories. Having a sweet tooth in Neolithic times was a great thing! You were likely to have more energy, and if you were really lucky and were able to eat enough naturally occurring sugar, you might even be fortunate enough to build some fat for lean times. And there would surely be lean times later on. That was just life.

Of course, we all know what happened. Our ancestors, led by their motivational networks and regular dopamine hits, figured out how to create a constant flow of sweetness. We cultivated plants with sweet flavors, applied our farming strategy, and provided ourselves with a stable source of sweet flavors that could be relied on. In our somewhat recent history, we have devised ways to extract sucrose from sugar cane and sugar beets, and we have satisfied our natural desire for the flavor by adding it to foods. Or in some cases, just making whole food groups out of sugar in general.

I can only imagine what it would be like to show an ancient man or woman the modern invention of "a candy store." The concept of "candy," a whole category of food unto itself, is the absolute opposite of what our Neolithic ancestors learned to seek out. It is infinitely more flavorful and infinitely less nutritionally valuable. Rather than finding a lifesaving caloric boost after several days of foraging and avoiding predators, we now give our children bags full of concentrated sugar to ingest as they sit on the couch and watch television.

I once had a conversation with a man who was walking the Appalachian Trail, a hiking trail that spans Springer Mountain in Georgia to Mount Katahdin in Maine (there are other extensions of this trail that reach further south and further north), a total distance of 2,200 miles (3,500 km). People from all walks of life dedicate months to walking the entire trail as a way to challenge their physical and psychological fortitude.

I was doing some overnight hiking with my father on the trail and was able to meet the sort of people who put their modern lives on pause for the chance to hike the trail in a single season. They literally live on the trail until they finish it. One such hiker shared with me that his secret was eating a candy bar when he felt down and ready to give up. The sudden rush of sugar filled him with energy to keep him motivated and moving. I remember his unkempt beard, his aroma of second-hand pot smoke, and his belt.

His belt was obviously purchased when he was significantly more ponderous. Its most pronounced wear-mark was three loops away from where he presently wore it. It seemed as though he was using far more calories in a day than he was taking in. Looking back on it now, his use of a candy bar was similar to our ancient ancestors' use of fruits and berries. It was a highly concentrated boost of sugar to fuel his body for the challenges of hiking long distances in the mountains.

Nature programmed us with preferences for salty and sweet foods because, in the wild, they are signs that a specific food is calorically dense or nutritionally valuable. They are not simply things that we like; they are internal guides for survival in the natural world, a world that we no longer live in. Yet, they still speak to us every time we choose what to eat for lunch. Yes, that question that people ask one another before going on a date, "Where would you like to eat?" is laughably modern. I can only imagine the look on our ancient ancestors' faces if we time traveled back with that question.

Eat? The answer is, yes. Yes, I like to eat. Where? I like to eat wherever the food is, please.

Our craving for fats—which contain nine calories for every gram, as opposed to four calories per gram of carbohydrate or protein—also continues to guide our choices. I love a good steak, likely because it is a great source of fat and sodium. And yes, the protein value of beef is impressive, but talk to any vegan and you will find out more than you wanted to know about the protein value of plants. What most plants lack—and what makes a slab of red meat so attractive to our biology—are fat and sodium, not just the protein.

Our bodies evolved during a time when a lack of calories was a daily struggle. Now, for most of the us in the West, not only have we solved that problem, we have handed down a life of obesity to our children. The National Health and Nutrition Examination Survey conducted research of American children and adolescents between the years 1971 and 1974 and found that 4% of children and 6.1% of adolescents were obese. More recent research by the same organization done from 2007 to 2008 reports that in the United States, 19.6% of children and 18.1% of adolescents are obese.

In solving the calorie problem, we have created a whole host of modern problems, most of which stem from the question: how will I convince myself to move more and eat less? As I am writing this, it is estimated that a human being somewhere in the world dies every seven seconds due to diabetes. This is based on a study published in *The Lancet* in 2011.

Chapter 5.

The Voice of Our Neolithic Grandma

It is important to put all of this into perspective. All of our drives and motivations come from countless years of human survival. We inherited a drive to solve problems, to eliminate uncertainty, and to seek out specific nutrients. We inherited them from our ancient ancestors because they were tools that provided them with the edge to survive and adapt. There is nothing wrong with you when you worry about what will happen tomorrow and wish you could eat chips and ice cream all day. You read that right, but read on. I'm not telling you to go to the fridge to have an ice cream party.

The reality is that you are a human, the same make and model as our ancient ancestors who lived a life of uncertainty in a world of scarcity. You are programmed by the hands of evolution to live in that world, not the modern world into which you were born. Humans are still naturally suited for life in the Neolithic era, not the 21st century. There is a clear disconnect between biology and modern life. Your sugar cravings, your proclivity for fatty cuts of beef, your tendency to worry, your anxiety; they are all there to help you survive. They are subprograms within your incredibly complex being, passed down through generations to help you. They are trying to help you, even though it seems, in today's world, that they are the root of all of our problems. This mismatch of drives and environment is a challenge that humans in the modern world share.

All those who came before us have also left us with the gifts of civilization, the products of their sleepless nights and anxieties. Some of them invented the wheel; others invented the modern mattress. All of them were driven by the internal need to mitigate the dangers of uncertainty while attempting to benefit from exploring the options that uncertainty brings. Driven by cravings for nutrition and sustenance, encouraged by the motivational network's dopamine hits, our ancestors changed the world. And here we sit, the beneficiaries.

But now that the world has changed, our old programming does not serve us as well as it once did. The cravings we share, in addition to the world that our ancestors created, can lead us to obesity, heart disease, diabetes, addictions, and countless other maladies if we do not take control of them.

Our impulses and drives are not trying to harm us. They are trying to help us survive. These impulses are your ancestors' loving messages, transmitted though time from one generation to the next through the conduit of our DNA. It is a beautiful and humbling thing to consider when you stop to think about it.

But on the other hand, there are times when grandma's advice simply doesn't apply to your life, right? It's not grandma's fault that she's a little out of touch. Things were different in her day! It doesn't mean she doesn't care about you when she gives you the outdated advice. She's just out of touch. That's all.

Just think about how out of touch your Neolithic grandmother would be, and now you have a perfect framework to understand some of your inner drives. Every impulse that we described before is the voice of your Neolithic grandma, trying to give you advice from her vantage point in ages past. I'm sorry, Neolithic Grandma, I shouldn't worry about tigers in the bushes, and I shouldn't eat every gram of fat, sugar, or salt that I find. I know you love me, Neolithic Grandma, but you just don't understand the world that I live in. Thank you for all that you have done for me, and thank you for the loving advice.

For most of my life, I was a Neolithic Grandma's boy. But there comes a time when we have to take responsibility for our own lives as they exist in the world in which we live, just like our Neolithic ancestors did. Even if we stop taking their advice, we can honor them by adapting to our modern world as they did theirs.

Perhaps our greatest challenge, as modern humans, is to understand how our bodies and minds work so that we can learn to live healthily in this world. This means learning to replicate the stresses in which our Neolithic grandmother lived without throwing away all of the benefits that we enjoy as modern humans. And this means that we cannot ignore the strange fact that we as a species require exercise, which often causes us discomfort. We also have to come to grips with the impulses that we naturally have, ones that our modern world have made all too easy to follow. We have to learn to take control of our eating habits rather than following our impulses to a life of obesity and poor health. For a human to thrive in the modern world, it is important to understand that there is a very real disconnect between the voice of our Neolithic grandmother and the modern world.

The Bridge Between Our Primal Programming and the Modern World

Of course, intellectually knowing why we are drawn to behave in certain ways doesn't necessarily mean that we will break free from these behaviors. Ask any addict. And here I don't necessarily mean a drug addict like I once was. You can ask someone who is addicted to eating sugary foods or living a sedentary lifestyle (okay, I was addicted to those things too…). In the modern world, we are aware that we should exercise and eat healthy foods, but simply knowing does not always lead to doing.

The same can be said for dealing with our dopamine feedback loops. We know that rumination doesn't solve anything, but we do it anyway. We live lives of anxiety and suffering that are completely created by our own thoughts, quite literally, a living hell.

We have gyms to provide us with the exercise we need, and we have grocery stores full of nutritious foods to help us feed ourselves in a healthy way. So, how do we take control of our anxiety? How do we learn to silence the chatter and reclaim our minds? We need a tool to bridge the gap between our primal programming and the modern world in which we live.

For me, there has been nothing more beneficial than the practice of breathwork, and I have seen breathwork's profound impact in the lives of my friends, family, and clients. When we practice breathwork, we practice taking control of ourselves in the most fundamental way. You can go without water for three days, and you can go without food for three weeks, but our breath is something so fundamental to life that we can never stop for longer than a matter of minutes. In the chapters that follow, I will explain to you how taking control of your breath will enable you to take control of your mental and physiological state, putting you in a position to make better choices and take control over your impulses. You will learn to interrupt the dopamine feedback loop and take back control of your thoughts. Breathwork doesn't do the work for you, but it is a powerful tool that you can use as you work on yourself.

But before we begin the next chapter, I want to give you the challenge that I give to my college freshmen, the words of Socrates, that "an unexamined life is not worth living." Now is a good time to examine your life. What impulses do you want to learn to control? How often do you find yourself stuck in a dopamine feedback loop? How often do you feel a generalized anxiety without even knowing what is causing it?

Take some time to think about the ways the disconnect between your primal programming and the modern world causes problems in your mood, in your outlook on life, in your relationships.

An Unopened Gift

Now get ready to open one last part of your inheritance. A powerful tool that your ancestors have left you, and a practical guide to use it. Congratulations on your inheritance! First let's learn about how our mental and physical state work, how modern life often conflicts with our programming, and how our breath can be used to give us control.

Chapter 6.
Introduce Yourself to... Yourself

Conscious control of breathing is an ability that only humans have. For all other creatures on earth, respiration is an automatic process governed by the autonomic nervous system. This is an ability that we usually take for granted. Most of us are unaware that this ability, conscious breathing, is so rare on planet Earth. When you take your dog out on a run, you are the only one who can decide to hold your breath, to breathe through your nose or mouth, or change the speed of your breathing.

The Autonomic Nervous System

To understand what is possible through breathing, it is essential to understand what the Autonomic Nervous System (ANS) does and how it governs various aspects of our physiology. The ANS is a system that governs things like heartbeat, blood glucose levels, circulation, and yes, among other things, breathing. As implied by the name, the ANS works automatically, without a need for our conscious control. This is good, because if it did not work auto-matically, we would have to remember to beat our heart, digest our food, and somehow consciously constrict or dilate approximately 60,000 miles of blood vessels in our body.

For humans, the ANS can be influenced consciously, but it is naturally influenced by what is generally called "bottom-up influence." That is to say that your ANS is connected with every other part of your Central Nervous System and is privy to a whole host of information. These are environmental cues, such as temperature, daylight, and situational cues. Your ANS receives this information and activates or deactivates systems within the body accordingly. The effect that this has on the body and its functions is as profound as it is ancient. To illustrate the way your Autonomic Nervous System was designed, let's go back in time to what your life would have been like for the vast majority of human history.

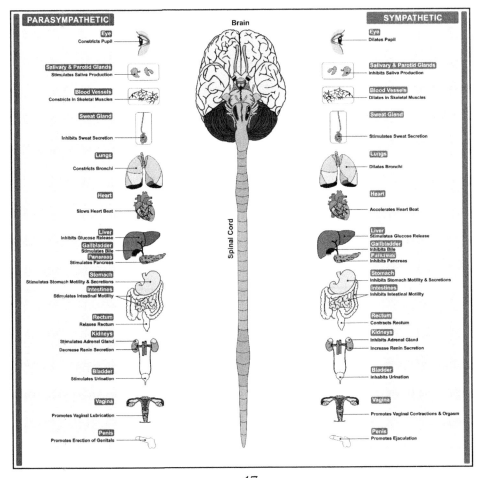

As a prehistoric human, you don't really have a profession like we think of them today. You are a Swiss Army Knife of a human. You are responsible for all aspects of your survival in a hostile world, full of things that have teeth and claws who are just as hungry as you are.

Among your many tools for survival is your Autonomic Nervous System. See the chart on previous page for a short list of what your Autonomic Nervous System will do for you depending on its state.

You wake up in a safe place. Let's just call it a cave, since that is probably the height of home building technology for your time. But, after you wake up, your stomach tells you that you need to fuel your body. It craves calories. Lots of calories. So, you look around your cave, and since your cave is not equipped with a refrigerator, you know that the only way to feed your hunger is to go out into the wild.

As you leave your cave, you are immediately in danger. That's fine, because your Autonomic Nervous System is there to help you. Without you even needing to think about it, your vision adjusts, your blood glucose increases, your breathing becomes more active, and your muscles become full of this oxygen and glucose rich blood. Things that you don't need for immediate survival—like your digestive system and your reproductive system—are inhibited, shutting down to allow for maximal energy flow to the systems that are most needed. You have entered a Sympathetic State, often referred to as the state of "fight or flight." Your state is perfectly adapted to the uncertainty of the situation. Dopamine hits encourage you to seek out and eliminate danger, and at the same time, you are poised to adventure into the uncertainty of the wilderness for the opportunity to discover advantageous opportunities (in this case, food).

Your sense of smell is heightened when you are in a sympathetic state. Did you know that? Well, you don't have to know it. It is automatic. As you traverse the wild landscape, your senses are heightened to help guide you to your prey and to help you avoid predators.

What's that? You glimpse a tasty looking antelope in the distance. With stealth and the undying hopes of having your next meal, you stalk the creature. But you aren't alone. Your tribe engages in this hunt together, and when all is done, your tribe distributes the parts of the antelope according to pecking order. Great, you have your rack of antelope on your back, fresh with blood dripping down your sweaty back.

You make your way back to your cave, careful to avoid attracting the hungry gaze of any predators that might be lurking in the unseen places.

When you get back to your cave, your autonomic nervous system, sensing that the situation has changed, begins to change your state from a sympathetic state to a parasympathetic state, also known as "rest and digest." Your autonomic nervous system detects environmental cues that inform it that you are in a safe place. You are in a familiar place, away from the uncertainty that surrounds you when you hunt. Your body and mind begin to relax.

Your muscles no longer bulge with blood as they did on the hunt. Instead, your digestive system, anticipating a feeding, begins to kick on. Your mouth waters as you roast your meat in your prehistoric kitchen, equipped with an open fire and a primitive version of a rotisserie. Your senses are not as sharp as they were when you were in the wild. Your breathing and heart rate have slowed down. You are relaxed.

Did you meet a special someone in the tribe earlier? In this parasympathetic state, you are now fully capable of using your reproductive organs too. Perhaps the freshly cooked antelope is just the first course in your prehistoric version of a dinner date.

That night, you can sleep deeply and fully. Your body is able to digest the food that you consumed and use it to repair the damage from the day. Injuries heal, muscles repair and grow stronger. You dream. You even get to deep sleep, the most recuperative sleep state, where there are no dreams at all. When you wake up, you feel rested and ready to do it all over again. All of this, without the mattresses that your future descendants will someday see advertised on television.

As a prehistoric human, your autonomic nervous system is perfectly suited for its environment. It senses environmental cues and makes changes accordingly. It knows when to become active, and it knows when to relax simply based on bottom-up cues from your environment. You thrive as an organism because you are in the right state to meet the challenges in front of you. And all of this happens without you having to be aware of it. As far as you know, your body is simply doing what bodies do. And this frees you up to focus on the world around you, building your spear, avoiding dangerous situations, finding your mate, working your way up through the tribal pecking order. Your internal software is perfectly in tune with the world it is living in.

Fast-forward a few thousand years and the world is completely different. However, our autonomic nervous system is still working under the same assumptions, that you are living in the wild, that your life is a series of events that range from a safe cave and a deadly hunt, that you would never eat while you hunt and you would never hunt or have to run from a bobcat while you are in your cave. But guess what, that is exactly what the modern world is like.

Ancient Programming in a New World

Well, okay, we aren't literally running from bobcats in our homes (unless you live a life WAY more interesting than mine!). But psychologically, we are doing just that. When we are put into situations of stress, our autonomic nervous system tries to do us a favor. It says, "I guess it's time to either kill something or run away from something deadly, so let's get into the sympathetic state." You sense uncertainty, which activates your motivational network's dopamine response. But in reality, the stress that you feel in the 21st century is likely not a life-or-death situation in the most real sense. Perhaps you receive an unexpected bill or have an argument with your boss. These are stressors that we can perceive as a stimulus for sympathetic nervous system activation. We experience activation, and this keeps us in a stressed state and fills us with anxiety.

Of course, you might like to "rip someone's head off" in a figurative sense, but your trusty ANS doesn't understand these modern conventions. Your ANS is in your corner, supplying you with enough adrenaline, oxygen, and glucose to really get the job done. Some people talk about "going medieval" on someone, but your ANS is even more old school. It is equipping you with the tools to kill or escape. All the while, you are just having an argument with Tammy about politics.

Of course, in the modern world, we are subject to life or death situations all of the time, but other parts of our brain are so good at adapting that we can drive on a freeway at deadly speeds without even remembering our drive home. Tons of metal whiz by our eyes daily on streets and highways, and we just call it everyday life. Do you really think you are relaxing when you are driving in traffic? Do you think you are in a state of "rest and digest" when you pick up food in the drive thru window and eat it on your way back to the office? Of course not. That would be like your prehistoric self trying to eat and hunt at the same time. We know that our ANS powers down our digestive system so that it can power up your muscles for fighting or fleeing. You are in a quintessential modern predicament: not only is your double cheeseburger devoid of most of its nutritional value, you're not even in the right state to digest it.

We also invite bobcats into our bedrooms and living rooms every time we look at the news, check social media, or participate in activities that invite the stress of the outside world into our modern-day caves. This is encouraged by the dopamine loop, which promotes exploration and investigation, trying to solve uncertainties. You might check your social media to see that Sally just got divorced. Really? What happened there? Was she cheating on her husband? Wait—was he cheating on her? Maybe there was domestic violence involved. I better check the comments to learn more. Maybe I'll ask Sally's friend, Tammy. She'll know something.

And on and on we go, constantly mismatching our state with our lives. And sleep? Well, we know what happens to our sleep! That mattress that promised to put me right to sleep is no match for countless generations of evolution, reinforcing systems within my mind and body.

So, the bad news is that much of our internal programming is not conducive to modern living. And we, like our ancient ancestors, are unaware that these systems are running. But where our ancestors were blissfully unaware because their systems were adapted to their environment, our lack of awareness leads to suffering. Why can't we "shut off our brains," or get the sleep we need, or have enough energy to make it through the day? So, we turn to the best inventions and prescriptions we can find, and all too often, we find that they are still not enough. Or we discover that prescriptions cost money and usually come with side-effects.

But it isn't hopeless. There are things that we can do to intervene. Powerful things. Free things. This is where conscious breathing and the art of mindfulness become powerful tools in "upgrading" our ancient software to be better suited to live in the modern world.

Breathing Provides "Top-Down" Control

Research has been done on how breathing affects the body and mind for decades. In the *Journal of Neurophysiology,* a 2019 study titled "Breathing Above the Brain Stem: Volitional Control and Attentional Modulation in Humans" showed an increase in activity in the amygdala, insula, and cingulative cortex depending on the speed and pace of the breathing of the participants. These are parts of our brain that are involved in autonomic functions of the body, memory formation, learning, and fear. The study focused on three conscious breathing techniques that varied in speed and pace. This is just one of the many studies that demonstrate that something as simple as changing our rate of breathing can cause changes in our brain activity, and therefore influence our state in profound ways.

In a conversation I had with Dr. Otto Muzik of Wayne State University, he told me that this conscious control over our breathing is a result of a coincidence that occurred when humans evolved into speakers. As we evolved the ability to speak, the need to modulate our breathing naturally arose. Just think of the intricate qualities of speaking and try to imagine what it would be like if you did not have conscious control over how much air you were breathing in and out. Speaking would be impossible. As Dr. Muzik explained to me, conscious breathing also provides us with a top-down way to control our state.

He said, "This is because our brainstem breathing centers just happen to be very close to brain centers that regulate our moods/emotions (as well as to the brain centers that initiate the norepinephrine release that make us anxious) and by tweaking the neural firing patterns in our breathing centers, we are able to directly influence what happens in these other centers."

Thus, rather than relying on outside stimuli to shape our body's state, we can take control of our breathing and influence our most foundational network, the homeostatic network in the brainstem, which can change our mood and emotional state.

Chapter 7.

The Secret Window | How Breathing Works as a Two-Way Communication for Your ANS

Breathing, unlike other things controlled by our autonomic nervous system (such as heart rate or blood glucose level), is a two-way communication conduit between the conscious mind and the nervous system. It is not only affected by our state, it can be used to change our state. Like our ancient ancestors, our state ("fight or flight" or "rest and digest") is still affected by bottom-up influences such as our environment and situation, but we are also able to use our breathing to influence our state at will (top-down). The implications are incredible. This means that by modulating your breathing, you can influence your heart rate, your blood glucose, even your ability to use your sexual organs.

Let's do a quick experiment to demonstrate this point. I want you to think about a time when you were afraid. Maybe you were just cut off in traffic. Maybe you were being chased by a dog. Maybe you were about to get into a fist fight. Try to think of a time when you were really afraid. Think about how you felt in that moment. How were you breathing? Was it fast-paced or slow? Did you feel the need to breathe more deeply into your chest, or did you breathe into your belly? Through the nose or through the mouth?

If you were really scared, it is likely that you were breathing quickly, that your breaths were in your chest, and you might have been breathing through the mouth. This is an example of bottom-up regulation of your autonomic nervous system. You perceived a threat via your senses. The sympathetic state of your autonomic nervous system was activated (also known as "fight or flight" response), triggering a whole host of physiological changes (see the chart of the ANS). One of the changes that the autonomic nervous system evoked was a change in your breathing. You didn't have to think about it. Your autonomic nervous system switched into "fight or flight," and your body geared up for action. When this happens the need for cellular energy increases, meaning that you need more oxygen to fuel your mitochondria. Again, this is an example of how the autonomic nervous system automatically makes adjustments, and your breathing changes as a result.

I assume that you are not reading this book while being chased by a dog. It is likely that you are in a parasympathetic state, also known as "rest and digest." Take a minute to observe how you feel, your energy levels, your breathing pattern.

Now, using nothing but our breath, let's see if we can change states. Try to recreate the breathing pattern that you had when you were afraid, the quickened pace, the rising of the chest with each breath, the mouth-breathing. Go ahead, take a minute or two to breathe as if you are about to get into a fight or run from a rabid animal. Don't hold back.

Seriously! Try this! Don't read the next paragraph until you have completed the experiment.

So? Did you try it? Do you feel a change in state? Are you more alert? You might even feel a rush of energy in your muscles. If you do, you have just influenced your autonomic nervous system voluntarily. You've done what no other creature on earth can do. Simply by changing your breathing pattern, you have increased blood glucose, reduced circulation in your digestive tract, increased blood flow to your muscles, and quite possibly increased the sensitivity of your senses of hearing, seeing, and smelling.

Don't worry, you aren't stuck in "fight or flight." With only a very short amount of time spent signaling a sympathetic response to your body, the activation probably wasn't that strong. And now that your breathing has returned to a relaxed pace, your autonomic nervous system will go back to looking for cues from your environment to provide bottom-up regulation of your state. In other words, now that you are no longer consciously sending yourself signals via a conscious change in your breathing, everything is going back to an automatic control.

However, I hope this little experiment showed you the very real communication pathway that exists by way of our breathing. We have the capability to influence nearly every element of our physical and mental state by way of conscious, controlled breathing.

We will learn specific techniques and protocols later in this book that have been developed for just this purpose, but for now, take some time to observe the subtle (and not-so-subtle) changes that occur when you speed up or slow down your breathing. You could also do an experiment where you think of a time when you were very relaxed. How did you breathe? Try breathing like that for a minute or two and see if you can detect a shift to the parasympathetic state of "rest and digest." Your breath is the secret communication pathway.

When we use our breath to influence our ANS, very real changes in circulation, blood sugar, hormones, digestion, sexual organs, and other autonomic functions occur. We are literally able to tell our bodies to focus energy in these areas. And just think for a moment about that. Here in the USA, we allow drug companies to advertise prescription drugs. I didn't realize that this was not common in other countries until I had a conversation with a Dutch friend of mine about this topic. He was flabbergasted, and it made me realize just how strange it is that we allow such a thing here. But if you live in the USA, just think about how many prescription and over-the-counter drugs you see advertised for issues that are related to things regulated by the ANS: blood pressure, blood sugar, digestion, hormonal imbalance, anxiety, and who can forget all of the erectile disfunction advertisements? It is easy to focus only on one part of our body and forget that everything is connected, and everything is affected by your autonomic nervous system.

Interrupting Anxiety

Remember the dopamine feedback loop in our brains, and the resulting norepinephrine dump? Remember how they are meant to help us, but they often leave us in a state of anxiety? When we are in control of our breathing, we can influence our state of arousal. When we breath in a manner that sends the signal "I'm safe," we can start to hack into our dopamine feedback loop.

By modulating our breath, we can also avoid the anxiety that comes from the norepinephrine dump that so often accompanies our dopamine feedback loop. In fact, in 2018, researchers at Trinity College Institute of Neuroscience and the Global Brain Health Institute discovered that one can affect the levels of norepinephrine released in the brain simply by practicing controlled breathing.

The study focused on the locus coeruleus, the part of the brain that releases norepinephrine. Norepinephrine is a neurochemical that is involved with attention and focus, but when levels are too high, we can feel anxious and struggle to focus. The researchers tested the subjects' respiration, locus coeruleus activity, and the ability to focus and found that those who focused well had better synchronization in their breathing than those who focused poorly. They found that respiration is directly linked to locus coeruleus activity, and that one can reduce the locus coeruleus's activity by modulating the subject's breathing patterns.

We get to decide to take control of our state, and it is possible with something as simple as breathing. Notice I used the word "simple" rather than "easy." This is because taking top-down control of systems that originally evolved to be outside of conscious control requires a great deal of focus. But it can be done, and it has been practiced by humans for ages.

The Vagus Nerve

Another important player in this equation is the Vagus Nerve. When you breathe, you either stimulate or inhibit your vagus nerve. You don't have to be an expert on the vagus nerve to be an expert at stimulating your vagus nerve. You just need to under-stand some basic principles. The most important principle is that your vagus nerve is intimately involved in communication between your Autonomic Nervous System and your breath.

The vagus nerve is a cranial nerve complex that is modulated by breathing. One of its many functions is to relay relaxation from the Central Nervous System to the body. When we exhale, we encourage the vagus nerve to send signals to relax. When we inhale, we inhibit the vagus nerve from sending signals of relaxation. Research suggests that vagus nerve stimulation influences blood pressure, heart rate, mood, and inflammation.

There are many ways to stimulate the vagus nerve, but none are so readily available to us as breathing. Research has shown that slow abdominal breathing stimulates the vagus nerve and induces the parasympathetic state. Fast and shallow breathing inhibits the vagus nerve and puts us into a sympathetic state ("fight or flight"). Your vagus nerve is always listening, always reacting. When we practice breathwork, we practice training our natural state of breathing to stimulate the vagus nerve, since we should naturally desire to be in a relaxed state in the majority of situations in life. Practicing a proper breath wave, using proper posture, breathing through the nose at all times, and using diaphragmatic breathing are practices that specifically improve vagal stimulation. As you read this book, focus on slow, low breaths that are consistent in their pace. You'll stimulate your vagus nerve and create a relaxed state for yourself.

All of these things are interconnected in the complex and beautiful creature that is you! I have only briefly covered the physiological and neurological aspects of how breathing affects our state, but you don't have to be an expert on how breathing affects your state in order to be an expert at affecting your state with breathing. Simply knowing that these things exist puts us in a privileged position amongst humans. For most of human history, we only had our own experience to guide us, completely clueless as to what was going on scientifically. Thanks to modern science, we know beyond question that breathing plays an enormous role in our health and wellbeing. This isn't just speculation; it is hard science combined with thousands of years of human experimentation. If we breathe poorly, our health suffers; if we breathe well, we can improve our health.

However, even though breathwork has been validated with modern research, its use by the masses has been limited. How can this be? We all breathe! Today, we know that we need to exercise and cut down on salt and sugar. We know that we need to cut down on chronic stress and anxiety. Today people run marathons, compete in Mixed Martial Arts, complete Spartan races, and have a whole host of diet and nutrition options at their fingertips. But shouldn't our first training be breath training? Breathwork is thousands of years old, much older than exercise bikes and green smoothies. Why has the West only recently opened up to taking this fundamental aspect of human health seriously?

Chapter 8.

A Brief History of the Breathwork Movement in the West

PRANAYAMA

Thousands of years ago, the yogis of India believed that if they followed the eight branches of yoga, they could reach enlightenment. This is still a path that many follow to this day. No book that covers breathing should forget the fourth limb of yoga, Pranayama. Pranayama is a compound word in Sanskrit: "prana" translates to "breath" or "life force." And "ayama" translates to "control" or "lengthening." This is the oldest and longest-lived form of breathwork. It is mentioned in the Rig Veda, an ancient Indian text which dates as early as 1500 BC.

One could claim that all of breathwork is essentially pranayama. However, to relegate pranayama to breathwork alone is to forget the richness of the yogic tradition. Pranayama is not simply breathwork. On the surface, it is. But on the surface, yoga is also just stretching and poses. Pranayama is a deeply spiritual practice that involves controlled breathing. It comes with claims about what each breathing technique does for the body and for the spirit. It is, and has been, practiced by countless practitioners in the East for thousands of years. Many Westerners have been inspired by pranayama, and have applied controlled breathing to their lives, but I think it is important to point out that without the spiritual element, controlled breathing is simply controlled breathing, not pranayama. Pranayama was not commonly practiced by Westerners until somewhat recently. In fact, controlled breathing, in the West, has a spotty history.

In the West today, the study of how breathing affects the body is respected and commonly researched. It has not been this way for very long. While conscious breathing has been a long-lasting aspect of the yogic tradition, in the West, it has only recently begun to be used therapeutically. And those who have used it in Western culture were often ridiculed for doing so. This wasn't always without reason. Many of the earliest breathworkers in the West held beliefs or performed practices that were far outside of Western cultural norms. I present to you some of the major players in the rise of breathwork in the West. While not an exhaustive history, I think this will illustrate why I think breathwork has taken so long to gain acceptance in the mainstream.

Reichian Breathwork

Wilhelm Reich was psychoanalyst known for his controversial ideas and methods of treatment. He was a student of Sigmund Freud, and he became one of the most influential and controversial characters in the early days of psychology. Among his many controversial methods of treatment was Reichian Breathwork, which he developed in the 1920's. This form of breathwork was performed in a therapeutic setting with a counselor. The process involves adding deep breathing, body positions, and a focus on muscular tension.

Therapeutic discussions of past and present turmoil are inserted before, during, and after this breathing technique is performed. The goal of the breathwork is to release pent up stress and anxiety that the patient may be holding back. In addition to the breathwork, a therapist might apply pressure to a specific area of the patient's body or ask the patient to move into different positions that might help in releasing the built-up trauma.

Reich was so controversial in his practices and views that he was banned from the International Psychoanalytic Association in 1934. Reich's breathwork was not widely used or heard of outside of the world of psychology. However, today, Reichian Breathwork is still used by some counselors, chiropractors, and holistic health practitioners.

Rebirthing

It is difficult to paint a complete picture of the origin of breathwork in the West, but many people agree that its origins can be traced to the 1960s and 1970s, when the yoga movement, the New Age movement, and the psychedelic movement were dawning.

Lenard Orr is known as the father of breathwork in the West. He was the inventor of a technique now known as Rebirthing, a form of breathing that he invented in the 1960s and perfected in the 1970s. He claimed that his circular breathing rhythm could do practically everything, from curing the common cold, to curing migraines and even expunging stuck birth memories. He said in his book, *The Healing Manual*, that most terminal illnesses and mental disorders are caused from the trauma and stress of birth. He believed that his breathing technique could allow a person to relive the birthing process and repair the birth trauma, leading to a longer healthier life. This form of breathwork was first performed in a hot tub, but was later adapted to be practiced in a dry setting.

Lenard Orr also believed in physical immortality. He claimed to have met and trained under five immortals early in his career. He claimed that living life according to the elements would bring forth eternal life and based most of his message on the teachings he was given from the immortals, personal revelations, and the yogic traditions.

Rebirthing was promoted as a spiritual path that promised to raise a person's frequency, allowing a person to advance to ascendancy. Thousands of people from all around the world have practiced Lenard Orr's breathing technique, and there are countless stories of people who have benefited greatly from his practice of Rebirthing. On the other hand, I don't think it is a stretch to say that his New Age approach and grandiose claims about physical immortality were a big turn-off to most people during the late 20th century. Lenard Orr died in September of 2019 at the age of 82.

Liberation Breathing

Another notable pioneer in the field of breathwork is Sondra Ray, who was a contemporary of Orr and is known as the "Mother of Rebirthing." She pioneered a technique that she calls Liberation Breathing which was something that a person would learn after becoming very proficient with Rebirthing. She claims that Liberation Breathing can allow the practitioner to "receive the energy of the Divine Mother," and that "working with the Divine Mother energy makes everything about nine times more powerful."

Both Orr and Ray professed that they had met a spiritual character named Babaji, "an immortal avatar and yogi master." To fully understand Babaji, here is an excerpt from Sondra Ray's website, sondraray.com (as of 4/11/2020):

> Babaji, also named Sri Sri 1008 Bhagwan Herakhan Wale Baba, is an immortal maha avatar and yogi master ("avatar" means 'descent of the Divine into matter' without being born of a woman) babaji is an emanation of Divine Light, who, out of compassion, manifested in human form on earth to urge humanity to progress on the path of truth, simplicity, love and service to mankind. He is the power of the Eternal Father, Mother and Divine Child. He can assume any form He wishes and can change that form at any time. He is known as the historical Sada Shiva in Hindu religious literature. In fulfillment of ancient scriptural and prophetic predictions, He materialized a youthful body in a cave near the village of Hairakhan in the foothills of the Himalayas in 1970. There are Indian devotees who tell stories of this, and Yogananda wrote about him in the book *Autobiography of a Yogi.*

> Babaji was accessible for 14 years on his last visit in that body. And yet He has not left, because He does not come and go. He was, and is, omnipresent. His form is limitless and beyond the scope of time. He is the essence of all religions and transcends every belief. He teaches through vibrations and direct experience in a way that words can not express.

Orr and Ray travelled the world leading workshops, retreats, and talks. They authored various books on Rebirthing and Spiritual Self Mastery. Again, it is easy to see how this movement only attracted a specific kind of person. For the majority of people, the dogma attached to the breathing technique was enough to prevent them from ever trying it.

Holotropic Breathing

In the 1990's a new wave of breathwork was introduced by a husband and wife team, Stan and Christian Grof, who were trained in classic psychoanalytic therapy. The goal of Holotropic breathing is to induce a state of altered-consciousness to access parts of one's consciousness that are not normally experienced. Using prolonged sessions of hyperventilation, the oxygen supply is cut off from the brain, and the practitioner is said to be able to relive one's birth, access and address past trauma, and even access past-life memories. These sessions generally involve a "sitter," a person who sits with the breather while the session takes place. This "sitter" is in charge of helping to guide the breather through the process, at times offering encouragement, other times simply being a quiet observer, and even other times engaging in bodywork to help the breather to get the most out of the experience.

After the breathing sessions, participants are encouraged to draw visual representations of what they experienced. These representations are called "mandalas." They then have a group session where people are encouraged to show and explain what they drew on their mandalas. In these sessions, people describe experiences that range from colors and lights to reliving a rape in a former life. This form of breathwork has been practiced by hundreds of thousands of individuals across the world, and has been reported to be beneficial by countless participants.

Sessions of Holotropic Breathwork can be viewed on the internet. To an outside observer, these videos can appear incredibly disturbing. People writhe and shake; their faces wince in what seems to be extreme pain. People scream at the top of their lungs, and look and sound as if they are experiencing an exorcism. For most onlookers in the 1990's, this was likely a major turn-off. And while Holotropic Breathwork did not espouse the esoteric dogmas that Rebirthing and Liberation Breathing did, they were still full of extremely controversial topics such as past life regression, reliving birth traumas, and spiritual awakenings. While this form of therapy was and still is very popular, the vast majority of individuals looked at it as something too weird or scary to try.

Heart Math

In 1991, The Heart Math Institute was founded by Doc Lew Childre Jr., who was the son of the famed Grand Ole Opry singer, Doc Lew Chilre Sr. The Name "Doc" was a nickname that he inherited from his father; he is not a doctor. After developing some health problems, he looked for alternative methods for finding health. He realized that stress played a major factor in health, and sought ways to address the issue. The Heart Math Institute (HMI) has since conducted research into what they call "heart coherence," which is the measure of synchronicity between the heart's rhythm, the respiratory system, and other various biological systems. The HMI has used a variety of methods to improve the health of their practitioners, including biofeedback and focused breathing exercises. They focus on autonomic control, heart rate variability, and polyvagal theory to produce heart coherence to harness what they claim is the intelligence of the heart to lead a better and healthier life. Over the decades, they have produced music that is said to calm a person into a state of relaxation, and biofeedback devices to help people find the state of coherence. Today, practitioners can purchase these devices, which will work with a smart phone, and be led into a guided meditation that emphasizes the importance of relaxed breathing and emotional states that facilitate health.

The Heart Math Institute is respected by some and laughed at by others. Like the previously described breathing techniques, Heart Math has been practiced by thousands of people from all around the globe, and countless people have shared incredible life-changing results. However, unlike Rebirthing, Liberation Breathing, and Holotropic Breathing, Heart Math is pretty boring for some people. It does not make grandiose claims or provide visions or intense sensations of euphoria. It offers subtle changes that accumulate over time, and as a result it is still only adopted by a select group of practitioners.

Breathwork in the West was sporadic, and generally only interested people on the fringes. While Heart Math does offer a significant amount of science to back their claims, even now, it has not yet become a household name. It was this inconsistent, unreliable dynamic into which another person stepped. His work would change the history of breathwork and alternative healing practices, forever. His name is Wim Hof.

Chapter 9.

How I Found Breathwork Through Wim Hof

One day, I was scrolling on the internet and stumbled across an article titled "Learn to Influence Your Immune System Consciously." I automatically said to myself, this seems like some "woo woo" nonsense. What kind of moron would read such a thing?

So, of course, I clicked on the link and read the article.

I expected to read the article, pass judgement on the content, and go about my life. But it didn't go that way.

If you've not heard of Wim Hof, also known as The Iceman, you may be surprised that such an individual exists. Wim Hof has done what most people believe to be - not only impossible, but even supernatural.

He is best known for his world records with ice. He stood in a glass case of ice cubes, wearing nothing but shorts, for almost two hours. And he has done these feats multiple times, breaking his own record each time by one minute. His last record was one hour and fifty-six minutes.

Of course, like the goof that I am, when I met him later in person, I had to ask him, "why didn't you just do 2 hours flat?"

He looked at me with a smile, and said, "Maybe next time."

The source of his abilities? A health routine he calls, The Wim Hof Method, which consists of a breathing exercise, regular cold exposure, and mental focus. Using this method, he made the first claim that I had ever heard that we are capable of influencing our autonomic nervous system.

Wim Hof | The Radboud Study

In 2012, Hof made the claim that he could influence his autonomic nervous system, and thereby influence his immune system simply by using his Wim Hof Method.

Scientists at Radboud University conducted a test on Hof to test his claim. They injected him with an endotoxin of e coli, a dead fragment of the bacteria cell that will still elicit the innate immune response, replete with its usual symptoms of fever and extreme nausea. While the control group experienced all of these symptoms, Hof, practicing his breathing technique, was able to suppress his innate immune response, leaving him symptom free except for a small headache that he reported having.

Of course, this could be written off as Hof simply being a genetic anomaly, but he insisted that what he was capable of doing, anyone could do by practicing his method. So, the experiment was repeated by Radboud University in 2014 with twelve volunteers being trained by Hof to practice his Wim Hof Method. The twelve were subjected to the same endotoxin, and they were able to do the same thing. While the control group suffered for 24 hours, those who were practicing Wim Hof Method displayed fewer pro-inflammatory markers and fewer symptoms overall. The landmark study put Hof on the world stage as someone who had stumbled upon a way to influence the autonomic nervous system and, as a result, the immune system.

Many people have made claims like this in the past, but what made Hof different was that he was willing to go to science, and his results were observable in other people, not just himself. The significance of the study was expressed by Pikker and Cox in their article in *PNAS* titled "Voluntary activation of the sympathetic nervous system and attenuation of the innate immune response in humans" in the following way:

> Hitherto, both the autonomic nervous system and innate immune system were regarded as systems that cannot be voluntarily influenced. The present study demonstrates that, through practicing techniques learned in a short-term training program, the sympathetic nervous system and immune system can indeed be voluntarily influenced. Healthy volunteers practicing the learned techniques exhibited profound increases in the release of epinephrine, which in turn led to increased production of anti-inflammatory mediators and subsequent dampening of the proinflammatory cytokine response elicited by intravenous administration of bacterial endotoxin. This study could have important implications for the treatment of a variety of conditions associated with excessive or persistent inflammation, especially autoimmune diseases in which therapies that antagonize proinflammatory cytokines have shown great benefit.

This is the most famous study that Wim Hof has ever been involved with, and it set him apart from so many other breathworkers that had come before him. He wasn't simply making claims, he was proving them in the laboratory.

Instead of passing judgement on the article, I became incredibly interested in learning more about this man, his method, the power of breathwork, and what a cold shower could possibly do for my health. I started practicing his method, and before I knew it, I was hooked.

My Deep Dive Begins...

My sister is a Yoga instructor. I kept telling her about Wim Hof Method so much she told me I should try to become a Wim Hof Method instructor. Of course, the only problem was that there were no Wim Hof Method instructors in the whole world at this time. Well, there was only one, Wim Hof himself, and he was all the way in the Netherlands. He led excursions in Spain and in Poland, and as far as I could tell, no one else was qualified to teach his method.

So, I asked a question on a message board, asking if I went to a Wim Hof excursion, would that make be qualified to teach Wim Hof Method? It was a shot in the dark, but I got a response. It was from a European ice swimmer who was going to be in the first class ever to be certified to become a Wim Hof Method Instructor, and she said there would be a European Class and an American Class. Wim Hof was going to come to America. And he would be certifying the first ever group of instructors to teach his method.

So, I bought a ticket to Los Angeles and flew out for the first of two major training modules. There, I met Wim Hof for the first time. I could hear his distinct voice long before I was close enough to see him. I remember glimpsing him in the distance as I walked to the building where the training would be held. He spotted me walking in the distance, as I ducked around a tree conspicuously, trying to see his face more clearly. He looked back at me.

"Wim Hof? Is that you?" I asked loudly as I approached.

"There is only one of me!" He yelled back in a thick Dutch accent. "Nobody else out there as crazy as me!"

I also became acquainted with dozens of other people who were also joining this new world of breathwork and cold exposure. There were doctors, yoga instructors, martial arts experts, personal trainers, and people from lots of other walks of life. We were part of a movement that had only just begun to take hold in the USA. It was an exciting feeling.

After that weekend in 2016, training with Wim Hof, I went home and began training for the final Master Class. I also began researching everything I could find about how breathing affects the mind and body.

Examining Hof's Breathing Technique

When I first discovered Wim Hof and his method, I was under the impression that his breathing technique was practically a magic trick, that somehow this specific number of deep breaths and the breath holds somehow unlock aspects of the human mind and body, like a combination lock or an incantation. I didn't know any of the information that I covered in the previous chapters at this time, so I made a mistake that I want you to avoid: I focused too much on following a specific protocol and too little on observing, listening, and experiencing. I was looking for a combination or an incantation when I should have been observing the connection between my breath and my mind and body.

Hof claims that he discovered his breathing technique in nature, that it isn't a technique that he learned from books or anyone else. This was and still is widely disputed, but after closely studying all the breathing techniques that I have been able to find, I've never seen the exact same protocol used in the exact same way. This does not mean that there are no other breathing techniques that are similar. And this does not mean that he was not aware of the power of breathing and its influence over the mind and body when he developed his protocol. Hof is a master yogi, so he was surely aware of pranayama.

Thousands of years ago yogis and mystics were experimenting with breathing, and they were able to discern that the way we breathe can affect the way we feel. Without the guidance of scientists or even the formal knowledge of the brain or the systems in the body, they were able to do this through self-observation and trial and error, combining their acquired knowledge over the years and giving future generations the fruits of their self-exploration.

What I realized about Wim Hof was that he did the same thing as the ancient yogis. He observed the subtle and profound changes that breathing caused and consequently added to the body of knowledge of breathwork. While I have learned a lot from Hof, I think the greatest lesson is that one can learn a great deal simply by paying attention and experimenting. Yes, we are all capable of practicing his protocol, but we are also capable of discovering incredible things about ourselves simply by applying our curiosity and willingness to listen.

Breathing with Hof

My hands were clenched, the muscles in my arms were flexing without my asking them to. I could barely feel face. But the little bit of sensation I had in my face informed me that I would not be able to control the muscles in my face if I tried.

Alongside my fellow instructors-to-be, I had just engaged in 30 minutes of the most intense breathwork I had ever experienced. Up to this point, I had been practicing Wim Hof Method for over a year, diligently practicing breathwork daily, but I had never experienced such an incredible session of breathwork. Hof and his assistant, Kasper van der Meulen, had just taken us through an extended deep breathing session, something they called DMT Breathing. I was experiencing an altered state, and it felt amazing.

As I began to re-align myself with the rest of the world, I could hear some of the others in the room who had just experienced the same thing. Some of them were laughing. Some crying. Most of us were simply smiling with closed eyes, taking in the experience that we had just been privy to.

I felt a sense of oneness with everyone who was present, a sense that I was a part of everyone and everything around me, and that everyone and everything around me was a part of me too. A sense of wholeness. There was a mood of understanding that swept over the group, and everyone seemed compelled to hug and share smiles of compassion.

Training under Wim, we were led through deeper and longer sessions of breathwork many times. These sessions would go on for what seemed like an eternity sometimes. "Breathe!" Hof would demand. "Continue your breath, just be present," he would say.

And eventually, after what felt like days of nonstop deep breathing, he would instruct us to take a deep breath and squeeze into the head. What would follow was intense and profound. Each experience was different, and it seemed as though each experience was perfect for the moment.

I will never forget one such breathing session that Kasper van der Meulen led us through while we trained in the Rocky Mountains. After an intense session, I remember walking out of the cabin that we were collectively staying in. The world was bright and fuzzy, dreamy. As I walked out, I saw the mountains in the distance. The visibility was perfect that day. I remember looking at the mountains and feeling a sense of family with them. That all of creation was related, full of love, and open.

Of course, this might all sound strange to some readers. I will just say that breath can take you places you did not know you needed to go. To this day, I am still blown away that something as simple as breath can be used in so many ways. Not only can it influence mood, the ANS, and therefore a long list of bodily functions, it can launch us into states of being that we cannot normally experience. No drugs needed. Completely free of the worries of modern life.

Realizing the Relationship Between the Image and the Reality

Training with him in the Rocky Mountains, I got to see Wim Hof as he really is, without the mist of idolatry that I had once seen him through. I was starting to understand the mechanisms of breathing and cold exposure better than ever before, just as I was starting to see Wim Hof as a human rather than some kind of guru. I was also starting to understand that, once you understand the fundamentals of breathing and cold exposure, it is really easy to apply them to improve your life. It isn't anything mystical. If anything, it is practical once one understands the principles of these two modalities.

I completed the Wim Hof Method Certification training and started travelling all around the American Midwest, training hundreds of people in Hof's techniques, keeping up with the Hof community, and playing a role in bringing breathwork and cold training to the USA. I have had the pleasure of working with Hof multiple times since training under him in 2016, presenting and assisting him in leading Poland excursions. I count myself very fortunate to have been able to train directly under Hof so early.

In this way, teaching the Wim Hof Method was the beginning of my deeper education in how breathing affects the body and mind. It wasn't good enough to simply understand the science of the Wim Hof Method, or to simply focus on this one technique. I had to learn about how it all worked.

Wim Hof was My Gateway Drug

The concept of a "gateway drug" became popularized in the 1980s to identify specific drugs that were perceived as dangerous simply because they might lead a person to try other drugs. For me, Wim Hof was my "gateway drug" into the world of breathwork. After practicing Wim Hof's breathing technique, I began to search for other techniques to learn. I was constantly learning something new, taking courses, attending workshops and seminars, reading books, learning from other breathworkers, and experimenting with my own breath.

Before long, I was coaching athletes, visiting college classrooms, and leading breathing classes for healthcare workers, teachers, recovering addicts, and other seekers of better health and wellness. What started with a click on an unbelievable article about Wim Hof led me down a journey to becoming a professional breathworker.

Chapter 10.

Communicating with the Body | The New World of Breathwork

Where I once thought Hof had stumbled onto some kind of secret code through his specific eponymously named method, I now realize that he was using the modalities of breathing and cold exposure to send the body signals. So much of the verbiage around breathwork and alternative medicine has to do with listening to the body and speaking to the body, concepts that are usually expressed with the same reverence as prayer. But all that Hof was doing, all that anyone can do, is interact with one's body and mind, and with the right stimuli, one can influence the body and mind in ways that might seem too good to be true.

When we talk about communicating with the body and mind, it leads to a lot of misunderstanding. We can put this "communication" concept in a different perspective. We intuitively understand that a sedentary lifestyle with an overabundance of sugar, salt, and calories harms our bodies. We understand that when we slouch or look at our screens all day, we affect our posture. These are communications with our bodies and minds. We are providing signals to ourselves on a level that is deeper than language.

A Remedy for the Negative Effects
of the Modern Human Condition

Breathwork is a method of communication with our bodies and minds. It is in this way, that breathwork can correct the maladaptation between our primal selves and the modern world, the modern human condition that keeps us from fully thriving in modern times. Where we once could rely on "bottom-up signals" to determine our state, such as the safety of the cave to induce a state of "rest and digest" or the danger of predators to induce a state of "fight or flight," it is now our responsibility to make this determination. Once we do this, we can reclaim the health and vitality of our ancient ancestors while still living in the modern world.

"Bottom-up signaling" (environmental signals that inform the Autonomic Nervous System to create state changes) will always be a part of our internal wiring, and a whole host of biohacking devices have been invented to recreate these natural signals. You might have a pair of blue-light blocking glasses, which you might wear in the evenings to improve your sleep. One of the strange realities that we modern humans face is that modern indoor lights replicate daylight so well that they continue to send "bottom-up signals" to our nervous system that it is not time to go to sleep, that it is still the middle of the day. This has been shown to interfere with the modern human's natural circadian rhythm, all because we are unwittingly receiving a "bottom up signal" that it is daytime, and therefore not time for sleep.

So, it is important not to forget that we are constantly receiving "bottom-up signals."

Since breathing provides us with a way to consciously send signals to our Autonomic Nervous System, we can use it to take conscious control over our state rather than having to rely on external inputs. In this way, we are consciously controlling our state through breathing, reclaiming the benefits we inherited from our ancient ancestors. We can choose to use this communication pathway to increase energy or induce a state of relaxation. While we cannot always rely on our external world to provide the cues we once relied on to change our state from Sympathetic ("fight or flight") to Parasympathetic ("rest and digest"), we can use our breathing patterns to do this for ourselves consciously. What a great inheritance!

So, how does breathwork... work?

So, what most people want to know is two things:
1. How does breathwork work?
2. What can something as simple as breathing do for me?

The second half of the book will answer some of these questions, but for now, I want to equip you with a very important tool for understanding breathing and its connection to your health.

The Autonomic Nervous System Decoder Ring

A Decoder Ring was a cheap plastic toy that used to come in kids' cereal boxes to entice snot-nosed kids (like me) to ask their parents to buy their brand of cereal. They could be used to decipher simple coded messages with your friends, and the idea was that you could send special messages that the grown-ups could not understand. Of course, that was assuming that you had something to say that was worth encoding. Let's face it, there are not a lot of things that 7-year-olds have to say to each other that really need to be encoded. I think the usual message I sent to my friends was something like: "You eat boogers."

But the tool that I want to equip you with right now is something like a decoder ring, one that is capable of sending and receiving encoded messages to and from your Autonomic Nervous System (ANS). And, while the second half of the book is dedicated to specific techniques and routines, the most fundamental element of breathwork depends on this tool of communication between your conscious mind and your ANS.

The Decoder Ring

Here is the foundational code of breathwork:

Breathe like you are nervous

ANS code for: create "fight or flight" state

Breathe like you are running

ANS code for: create "fight or flight" state

Breathe like you are sleeping

ANS code for: create a relaxed state

Breathe like you are safe

ANS code for: create a relaxed state

Do you see the pattern? Simply by changing our breathing patterns to match the state that we would like to inhabit, we can send the signal to the ANS to create that state. Changes in hormones, digestion, and circulation all follow because we have sent the message to the ANS. The ANS takes care of the rest.

This is why it is important to know what healthy breathing looks and feels like. We are often so removed from healthy breathing patterns that we are not really sure what it looks or feels like to "breathe like you are safe." And don't worry. We are about to cover what a healthy breath looks and feels like.

Chapter 11.

Breathing as a Tool for Life

You don't have to subscribe to any one breathwork method or protocol. The bigger takeaway is that human beings can influence their health and wellbeing using conscious breathing. These are not mysterious techniques that require a belief system or a devotion to one person or cause. The connection between breathing and wellbeing is simply part of the human experience that the masses never understood.

Another reality is that no matter what you do, you ARE influencing your health and wellbeing with every breath you take. Whether you're conscious of it or not, you are sending signals to your body and mind via this pathway, and just as you can practice a breathing technique to encourage a specific state of mind, your daily breathing habits can put you into an unhealthy state, even without you knowing it.

Case Study: Breathin' Steven

Steven is worried about a deadline coming up. He imagines all of the awful things that might happen if he does not meet the deadline. His powerful human brain, fueled by lots of dopamine, feeds him an endless supply of scenarios and circumstances that he can't help thinking about. Consequently, his breath quickens. Even though he is sitting at his desk, his sympathetic nervous system is become active, as if he may soon need to physically fight off an unknown threat (in this case, he is perceiving the deadline as our ancient ancestors would perceive a predator). He doesn't realize that his chest has become more active, and he has started taking more breaths in and out through his mouth. *He* doesn't realize it, *but his ANS does.* Having received "top down" signals from his breath (quickened and nervous), the "fight or flight" state is reinforced, creating a feedback loop reinforced through breathing. The quickened breath creates an even more intense "fight or flight" state, which leads to even faster breathing. Eventually Steven realizes that he is breathing heavily. This frightens Steven, leading to an even deeper state of "fight or flight." Chest breathing, mouth breathing, and freaking out, Steven is unaware of how he got to this point and unaware how to interrupt this cycle.

People everywhere have experiences like Steven's. Sometimes they are caused by worry; sometimes they are caused by poor posture. For many, instances like the case above are so common that we simply believe that something is wrong with us because we are always nervous and anxiety ridden. We often look to pills, powders, and prescriptions for help. And in so many cases, the answer is something far simpler. Learn how breathing works, and you can use it as a tool.

Breathwork is Your Birthright

I believe that breath is the birthright of every human being. It's not just for athletes. It's not just for yogis. You don't have to be spiritual. You don't have to be athletic. And you can be both of those things if you want. It really doesn't matter what your "why" is. Learning to modulate your breath to control your physiology is a tool that has always been accessible to you, and now you have the choice to learn to use it. You come from a long line of humans who learned to adapt to their environment. And don't forget Neolithic Grandma! Her voice still calls to you, trying to help you survive. But when we learn to use our breathing, we learn to take control of our minds and bodies in a way that can override the impulses she speaks into our lives from the ancient past. We love you, Neolithic Grandma, but we have to learn to grow up, just as you did. We can take it from here.

My goal (and I assume your goal too) is to learn to interact with my body and mind in a way that produces the best life possible. I'm not concerned with being an immortal yogi or proving anything to anyone. I just want to be able to sleep at night. I just want to get the most out of my workouts. I just want to feel confident and secure. Basically, I want to equip myself with enough knowledge about how my mind and body work so that I can properly use them. After all, I know of no other way to live life than with my mind and body.

Honoring our Neolithic Grandma

Just as our Neolithic ancestors found themselves in a world that they had to learn to adapt to, we find ourselves living in the world of the 21st century. Modernity has many blessings, but as we have discussed, it is a significantly different environment from the one in which our species evolved. Strong impulses, voices within us trying to help us survive, often lead us to unwanted maladies that are only possible in the modern world. But now we know. And now we can adapt. We can learn to live in this new world that we inherited from our ancestors, honoring them by learning to thrive in this new landscape.

The rest of this book is dedicated to explaining how to make breathwork a part of your life. For our ancestors, the invention of physical tools was the edge that our species needed to thrive in a world without civilization. For us, we must learn to utilize a new set of tools to help us thrive in the civilization that our species has since built.

You don't have to believe any specific thing to practice any of these techniques. This is a practical guide. It is based on my personal research and experiences over the years, as well as scientific studies that I cite in the references section at the end of the book. May this guide serve you as you put together your own breathwork routine.

Chapter 12.

What is Breathwork?
Why Practice It?

As discussed in the previous chapters of this book, the term "breathwork" was first used in the West to describe a method for reaching an altered state of consciousness via breathing. The sessions were usually quite long, and they usually were meant for the purpose of reaching some kind of spiritual goal or expunging some kind of trauma. These forms of breathwork are still widely practiced today and are more popular now than ever before.

However, the term "breathwork" has grown to encompass a wider meaning. **Today, breathwork refers to any manipulation of breathing for any purpose**. Modern day breathworkers are not confined to a specific dogma, religious point of view, or purpose. You will still find breathworkers seeking a spiritual goal, but you will also find breathworkers who train elite athletes to recover faster from intense exercise and become able to get into "the zone" on command. You will find breathworkers who train CEOs to take control of their stress, to enhance their ability to focus, and to become more productive. While these same breathworkers might also be leading one workshop on Wim Hof Method over the weekend, on Monday night they might be teaching classes on how breathwork can enhance one's mediation practice, and Tuesday they might be coaching athletes to improve their endurance.

Breathwork is a wide and growing field that is still in its infancy. At the same time, it is a practice that dates back thousands of years. In this way, it has been with us all along, but only now has it been accepted and practiced in such a way that it does not have to be attached to any dogma or spiritual tradition. Much like meditation, breathwork gets its roots from our ancient ancestors who figured these things out without the help of modern science, and only now do we understand the basics of how the elements of breathing work.

A Rationale for the Style of Breathwork in this Book

This portion of the book is a guide to help you begin your own breathwork practice. While I will cover specific techniques that I use in my practice and in my breathwork workshops and classes, I want to start with the fundamentals. That way, with time and practice, you can experiment with creating your own techniques and protocols.

This guide is not meant to be exhaustive. It is not a list of all of the protocols and techniques in existence. That would be nearly impossible to create, and it would still require experimentation for you to figure out what works best.

No matter how your breathwork practice develops, there are a few truths that need to be recognized:

1. **Most breathing techniques are not explicitly scientifically proven to do a specific thing.** That is to say that there

is no team of scientists out there testing every breathing technique to determine what each one will do for the practitioner. Research takes time, resources, and interest, and frankly, not many scientists (or grants) are interested in researching breathwork. However, that is not to say that most breathwork techniques are not based in a scientific understanding of the way breathing affects the body and mind. This means that what I will be sharing with you in this book is generally based in science, even if the specific technique itself has not been studied.

We apply this way of thinking all of the time. For instance, based on our understanding of physics, engineers regularly build new machines to do specific things. They use a scientific understanding of how things work to build something out of the parts. In this same way, a modern breathworker can take what people have learned through science and through shared experience to create a breathing technique for a specific purpose. We are engineering an exercise for a specific desired outcome.

2. **Humans are different, and while there are many things that will work the same way for everyone, others will vary based on individual experiences.** This is true for everything that has to do with your body or your mind. This is the reason why five people can do the same exercise plan and eat the same diet, but they might all have different results.

Be prepared to listen to your own experience and tweak your practice to suit your own physiology.

3. **Experts disagree.** We see this in every field: experts disagree. One expert will swear by one method, and another will swear by another, completely conflicting method. And to make all of it even more confusing, they are usually both incredibly successful in getting results for themselves and their clients.

   To add to the confusion, I am going to be providing you with my own methodology that I swear by. And as I said before, since experts disagree, this means that something you learn from my guide might be something that, later in your journey, you completely disagree with. Just know that I warned you ahead of time! And know that I respect your eventual position. I hope I never see divided, rigid factions in breathwork. My hope is that breathwork will be a field where people can disagree, but at the end of the day they can admit that disagreements do not mean people can't still be friends.

4. **There are many names to breathing techniques, and this can be confusing too.** Many breathing techniques have names that originate in ancient Sanskrit. Others are only known by the ratio of inhale to exhale. There are sometimes styles of breathing that have multiple names. And all of this can be very confusing. In this guide, I will try to use the most common names, but I too have created names of my own that I feel are accurate descriptions, or easy-to-remember names for a given technique.

5. **Some breathing techniques are too dangerous to learn from a book.** Some breathing techniques really must be

learned from a trained professional, someone who can cover all aspects of safety and help you if you have a bad reaction. In my time as a breathworker, I have seen a rash of "breathworkers" (and I use the term in quotes to illustrate that they are really not fit to lead others) who lead people into very powerful breathing sessions without fully mastering what they are teaching.

These "breathworkers" usually learn from a free video or a hand full of workshop experiences, and because they were able to be led through the experience on their own, they believe that they are able to lead others. Most of these people have big hearts and want to share a profound experience with other people. They genuinely want to do good things for others. However, I've seen too many cases where these well-meaning novices lead people to have bad experiences, or even trauma. There is a level of risk that every seasoned breathworker takes on when leading people into altered state experiences.

Because there is so much variation in the human species, it is not uncommon for one person out of a group of ten to have a reaction that is different from the others, one that needs some extra attention. For this reason, I will only cover techniques that I feel are safe for everyone. And in the cases where there could be contraindication, I will provide warnings. Make no mistake, this guide will cover altered state breathwork, but I will leave it to you to find a teacher for the extreme techniques.

My purpose in sharing the principles and techniques in this guide is to provide you with the guide that I wish I had when I was beginning my practice, a practical guide to breathwork. I will cover the basic elements of breathing, how breathing allows us to influence our physiology and our state, and specific techniques that should create specific results for the majority of practitioners. These are techniques that I have not only researched and used myself, but techniques that I have led and continue to lead countless others in over the years as well. My goal is to provide you with a handbook to get you started, or to add to your breathing practice. These practices will hopefully provide you with valuable insights about how you can become a healthier and happier person through breathwork and proper breathing, and hopefully provide you with a path to a long healthy breathwork practice.

Chapter 13.

The Rules of Breathwork

There are three important rules to breathwork that I will explain below. I know no one likes rules, but I assure you that these rules are not here to fence you in or confine you. Following these three rules will help you get more out of your sessions and ensure a long and safe practice.

1. **Rule #1—Breath training is focus training.** If your goal is to use your breathing to control your state or to improve your athletic performance, you must learn to focus. Just think about what you are doing. You are trying to take conscious command of a system that is designed to be automatic and controlled fully through the sensory inputs from your environment. You can't expect to be flipping through your phone while you practice. You are trying to do something that is impossible for all other animals, and this means that you will need to establish a high level of focus and self-awareness.

   This rule also applies to learning the techniques of controlled breathing. There will be some techniques that are difficult to perform, especially at the beginning. Just as a baby doesn't have the neuromuscular control that adults have over their actions and movements, you will likely find that your diaphragm may feel like a muscle that you can't control with the same nuance as other muscles. This is normal, and things will get easier the longer you train yourself to focus on every micro movement. This will increase your mind-body connection with your breathing mechanism, and ultimately transform your everyday breathing into an efficient machine to power your cells.

2. **Rule #2—Leave your ego at the door.** When one begins a breathwork practice, amazing and life changing things can happen, but please remember that these changes can take time. They may vary from one person to another, and you shouldn't compare your results to others.' It is very common to hear accounts of how someone "cured" an illness or was able to take control over their body and mind in ways that seem incredible; then you look at your own practice and feel like a loser because you can't seem to do the same things despite following the same instructions.

Your journey is your own. And before you begin, just know that even those people who report amazing abilities have stumbling blocks and weak spots. I would love to tell you that the field of breathwork is empty of people who exaggerate their successes and downplay their failures, but the reality is that when humans are involved, you will always have these things.

Breathwork is a practice. This means we have to practice honing the skill. Those who find the greatest success will decide to enjoy the journey and understand that this skill will grow over time with regular practice.

3. **Rule #3—Success in breathwork depends on interoception.** We often talk about having five senses (sight, smell, touch,

taste, hearing), but the reality is that we have more than that. For instance, we have the sense of proprioception, which informs us of our orientation in 3D space. We also have the sense of interoception.

Put simply, interoception is the sense of the inner state of the body. It is something that I commonly refer to as "the inner voice." This sense is easy to use when we are sick, or feeling good, but we can also hone our sense of interoception to help us detect subtle changes within ourselves. The more we are in tune with ourselves, the better we can listen to the subtle signals that our body sends us. In effect, when we learn to use our sense of interoception, we are able to communicate with our bodies in ways that we cannot otherwise. This takes time and patience, but learning to use our sense of interoception is the key to a successful breathing practice. The techniques described in this guide are instructions that will only get you so far. When you have learned to use your sense of interoception, you will be able to make subtle changes to increase the effectiveness of every technique that you try.

Chapter 14.

Breathing Like a Baby

Conducting Your Personal Breathing Assessment

You might have heard the saying "sleeping like a baby." It means you're getting a great night's sleep, peaceful, restful, quiet. Of course, as a father, I often laugh at this saying, because I've lost a lot of sleep caring for a baby who would not go to sleep! However, it is true that when a baby sleeps, we adults have a lot to learn.

We are born into this world with some amazing programming. We are all born naturally perfect breathers, and if you have ever seen a baby sleep, you've seen perfect breathing in action. Babies naturally use their diaphragm. They breathe according to their real-time needs rather than out of habit, and their posture and mobility have not yet been altered by sitting in chairs, typing at desks, or looking at their phones. As parents, we spend our lives training them to be healthy adults, but we could actually learn a lot from them.

The first goal of any breathwork practitioner, before adding fancy techniques, should be to learn to breathe like a baby. Correcting breathing disfunctions and improving our daily breathing habits should be our first priority. And not just first, but constant. We cannot "fix and forget" our bodies. So, while you may fix breathing disfunctions and improve your technique, you will always have to work to keep the maladaptation of modern life from creeping in.

So, let's get started. Are you ready to breathe like a baby?

NOTE: In this section, I will describe some qualities of ideal breathing. To get the most out of your experience with this book, I recommend that you lie down and film yourself breathing. Perhaps get a buddy to film you from different angles, but at least get yourself from the side. I recommend doing this with a sports bra or without a shirt. You will want to be able to observe the subtle aspects of your breathing, so no hoodies or baggy clothes!

Assessment 1

1. **Lie down on your back. Relax.**
2. **Breathe naturally through your nose for 30 seconds.**
3. **Give your camera a "thumbs up."**

Assessment 2

1. **Now empty your lungs as much as you can and take a big inhale through your nose.**
2. **Repeat three more times.**
3. **Give your camera a "thumbs up."**

Assessment 3

1. **Now empty your lungs as much as you can and take a deep breath through your mouth.**
2. **Repeat three times.**
3. **Give the camera a "thumbs up."**

Assessment 4

1. Now begin to breathe full breaths quickly through your nose for about 20 seconds.

2. Give the camera a "thumbs up."

Assessment 5

1. Now breathe full breaths quickly through your mouth for about 20 seconds.

2. "Thumbs up" to the camera.

Assessment 6

1. Breathe as fast and fully as you can for 20 seconds.

2. "Thumbs up" to the camera.

Assessment 1- Your Resting Breathing Pattern

Assessment 2 & 3- Your Active Breath Wave

Assessment 4-6- Your Active Breath Wave with varied levels of intensity

Using the guidelines below, based on your Self-Assessment, you can try to discover your weak points. Exposing our weak points is key to resolving deficiencies and maladaptation.

General Goals for Breathing Patterns

The diaphragm is your primary breathing muscle. It creates a negative pressure in the thoracic cavity as it contracts, creating space for air. One of the primary goals in your breathwork practice should be the proper use of this muscle. Other muscles involved in breathing are the intercostal muscles between the ribs, the abdominal muscles, and some muscles in the neck.

Respiration should be a fluid action of these muscles working together, expanding the thoracic cavity, allowing for efficient breathing. The diaphragm contracts, negative pressure is created, the air rushes down into the lungs, filling the bottom lobes and then topping off with a full lung if needed.

Pull Every Breath Down Low

It is important to pull every breath down into the belly, sometimes called the "dantian" or the "lower dantian." One way of imagining this target is to take your hand and measure three finger widths down from your naval, and from there, two finger widths inside your abdomen (You are obviously only visualizing doing this last part). It doesn't really matter what you call it. What is important is that you pull every breath down with the diaphragm to this area and then expand the breath as if you are blowing up a balloon from this area.

Test it!

Proper breathing will be most observable in your belly, but it should also be felt in every other direction. One way to test if you are fully expanding your breath in the ideal target zone is to place your hands on the sides of your abdomen. They should both move outward. Then place your hands on your lower back. You should feel the breath here too. You should also feel the breath expanding downward into your pelvis (although, you won't feel that with your hands!). Your sides and back will not move as much as your belly, but they should be active in your deep breaths.

This low breathing facilitates ideal ventilation profusion, which basically means that you are pulling air into the lower lobes of your lungs where the majority of blood circulates. This allows you to take advantage of a greater gas exchange with every breath.

You don't need to know why it all works in order to take advantage of proper breathing. Just pull every breath down below your naval with every inhalation, expand out in every direction with your inhales, and prosper with every breath.

Ideal Resting Breathing Pattern

At rest, our breathing should be nasal and slow. Our chest and neck should not be active. Only the belly should be moving, and even then, it should not be very visible. When we are inactive or at rest, our need for air is at its lowest point, so our breathing activity should match. This breath is low in the abdomen, nasal, and at a slow pace. While the average person takes between 10 to 13 breaths per minute, the ideal pace of breathing when at rest is around 6 to 8 breaths per minute. (One breath includes the inhale and the exhale.)

The Active Breath Wave

When our physical demands increase, so should our breathing activity. When we are running, jumping, or doing other physically demanding activities, our need to exchange CO_2 and O_2 are much greater. Our muscles and tissue need an increased supply of O_2 in order to create ATP, and as our mitochondria use this O_2 during cellular respiration, CO_2 is produced in a much greater quantity.

We get rid of excess CO_2 by breathing it out. This increase in the need to exchange blood gasses causes us to need to breathe more fully and frequently.

The active breath wave, the ideal pattern of breathing for our most active times, begins low in the belly and then increases the volume of air by expanding the ribs and then filling the chest. It is a full and complete inhalation (belly, ribs, chest) followed by an exhale that follows the reverse pattern (chest, ribs, belly). For active breathing (whether it is exercise related or simply in an active breathing technique), this is the process that we will always follow. It is the natural mode of breathing when active.

The Paradoxical Breathing Pattern

There are some breathing techniques that use what is known as "paradoxical breathing," which is normally a bad thing if done within a natural setting. This is when we physically perform the breath wave in the opposite fashion from described above. In a full breath while using paradoxical breathing, the chest will appear to fill and the belly will be concave when inhaling, and then upon exhalation the belly will appear to fill. This kind of breathing is inefficient and can send the wrong signals to your ANS if it is your natural state of breathing. However, this style of breathing can be useful in some techniques, especially when working on focus and diaphragmatic control.

Checking Your Breath Wave

Most of us will have some point where our breathing pattern breaks down and goes into a dysfunctional pattern. So, don't beat yourself up if your breath waves were not ideal. Most people will do quite well in the first assessments and break down in the more intense breathing assessments. And if you passed with flying colors, don't get too cocky; lying down is the easiest position for breathing. Just because you could breathe with a perfect breath wave while lying supine doesn't mean that your breath wave remains perfect when you are sitting, standing, running, or doing whatever activity you like to do for fun. This assessment is a great way to check ourselves for dysfunctions, but now that you have completed this exercise, you can observe your breath wave in all of your other pursuits.

The good news is that even the worst breathing pattern dysfunctions are capable of being fixed completely. It just takes practice and mindfulness. Fortunately, we can take control of our breathing patterns and retrain ourselves to become more ideal breathers.

We Are Always Adapting, Always Training

If you look at a baby or even a toddler, you will likely see an ideal breathing pattern, set at an appropriate pace and using an ideal breath wave. Like so many things in life, our breathing patterns are subject to our habits. A toddler will usually have ideal posture and mobility too. It isn't until we humans learn to use things like chairs, screens, and start eating less-than-ideal food that we train ourselves into maladaptive patterns that result in a fundamental shift in the way everything else works.

Our posture affects our breathing; our breathing affects our state; our state affects our sleeping habits; our sleeping habits affect our eating habits; our eating habits affect our breathing patterns; our breathing patterns affect our state; our state affects our mood; our mood affects our actions; our actions affect our physical activities; our physical activities affect our posture; our posture affects our breathing; our breathing affects our state; our state affects… and so on and so forth.

When we approach our breathing, we are actually affecting our whole being, but it doesn't stop there. All of our actions, all of our inactions, all of everything we do, whether we are awake or sleeping, affects everything else. You can have a beautiful breath wave, but if your posture is poor, you will not get the most out of your breathing. Nor will you get the most out of exercise.

The body is constantly trying to serve you by adapting to suit the world that you are living in. This is why so many people in the world today suffer from Upper Crossed Syndrome and Lower Crossed Syndrome. Our bodies adapt to a life of sitting in chairs, typing at a desk, and looking at a downward angle at our cell phones. As I type this, I am contributing to my own posture, and as a result, I will need to do my best to counterbalance my posture to prevent maladaptation. However, I will tell you that it is very difficult to completely avoid the maladaptation that modern life brings, so don't get down on yourself if you suffer from these issues. Just remember to try and take regular actions to remedy your postural issues so that you can enjoy the benefits of a proper weight distribution and alignment within the body that you call home.

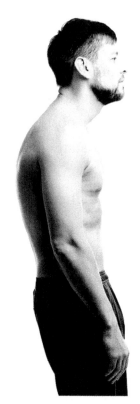 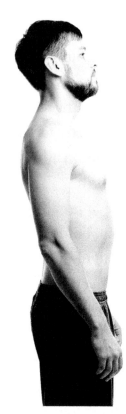

The image of the man on the left demonstrates both upper and lower crossed syndrome. These maladaptations are generally caused by muscle imbalances that result from patterns of living.

1. Upper-Crossed Syndrome is usually the result of inhibited neck flexors, rhomboids, and serratus anterior combined with tight pectorals, upper trapezius, and levator scapula. It causes the shoulders to droop and fall forward.

2. Lower-Crossed Syndrome is usually the result of weak gluteus maximus and abdominal muscles combined with tight erector spinae and iliosoas. This is also sometimes known as an anterior pelvic tilt.

These syndromes are usually caused by sitting in chairs and using a computer or a smart phone. The body is adapting to the life that it is leading.

One of the greatest strengths of yoga is that it improves mobility, posture, and breath control all together. One of the goals of a breathworker is to find balance within the body; this means being aware of your physical deficiencies so that you can address them.

The Ideal Posture

One reason for doing a breathing assessment in a supine (lying on your back) position is that it alleviates most postural issues from the equation. However, during the rest of your day, it is likely that you will need to be upright.

For ideal breathing, your goal should be to avoid upper-crossed and lower-crossed syndromes in favor of a neutral spine. When you have a neutral spine, your diaphragm and your pelvic floor will be in the ideal positions for the most efficient breath possible.

It is often helpful to think of the diaphragm and the pelvic floor as two ends of an accordion. We want them to be as parallel as possible, facing each other as directly as possible, avoiding inefficient angles that come with poor postural alignment.

When we add the element of a neutral spine to our breath wave, we are left with a smooth breathing flow.

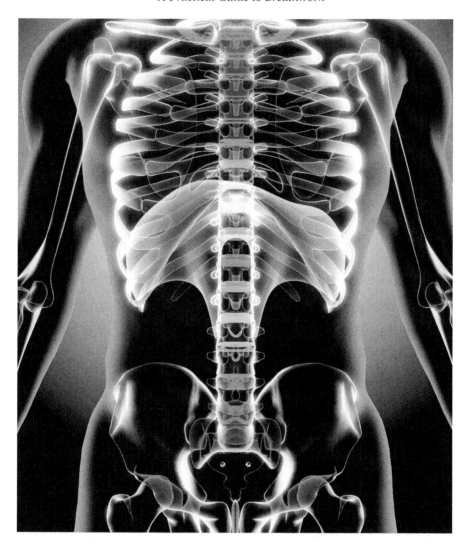

Nasal Breathing

Modern breathing specialists consistently talk about the importance of nasal breathing. This is for a good reason. Simply put, the nose is made for breathing. Nasal breathing not only filters the air, it moistens and thermoregulates each breath so that when the air reaches the lungs, it is at its ideal temperature, humidity, and purity for breathing. This makes breathing more comfortable and reduces irritation in the respiratory system, which encourages the alveoli to open up and function properly.

The nose also offers some resistance. Just take a deep breath through your nose versus your mouth and you can feel it. The ease in breathing that the mouth provides is why we often opt to use it, but the resistance offered by the nose engages the diaphragm and encourages a proper breath wave.

Mouth breathing encourages chest breathing, which is a sympathetic state trigger. In other words, when you engage in mouth breathing, it is likely that you are also engaging in chest breathing. Chest breathing, especially when done apart from a proper breath wave, is a signal to your ANS that you should change your state to "fight or flight." This is not the case with nasal breathing. When we are at rest and we want to benefit from the resting state, we must remember to breathe through the nose.

Nasal breathing has also been shown to increase levels of nitric oxide in the blood, a powerful vasodilator that plays a huge role in relaxing blood vessels and improving blood flow. When we do not breathe through the nose, we miss out on the benefits that this powerful molecule can provide. Simply put, our nose is the ideal breathing mechanism and should be used at all times, if possible.

Mouth Breathing

We are capable of switching to mouth breathing, and we naturally do this when nasal breathing does not allow us to meet the physical demands of intense activity. When we breathe through the mouth, we can increase the volume of air that we are able to move in and out of our respiratory system, increasing our capacity to rid our bodies of excess CO_2. There is nothing wrong with mouth breathing if done in the appropriate instances. However, mouth breathing can have negative impacts when we do it too soon with relationship to our physical demands or too often. The key is to delay mouth breathing as long as possible.

As stated above, breathing through the mouth encourages chest breathing and therefore is likely to send a signal to the ANS that we should switch states from the resting parasympathetic nervous system to the active state for the sympathetic nervous system. This is fine in short doses, but we are not meant to be stuck in the sympathetic nervous system. It is appropriate when we are sprinting, jumping, rowing, or fighting, but many people breathe through their mouths when they are typing at their desks, reading a book, or even sleeping.

Habitual mouth/chest breathing leads to:

1. **More anxiety in daily life.** Even though you intellectually understand that you are sitting at your desk, you are sending your ANS (and therefore every other part of your nervous system) a signal that insists that you are not safe, and that you need to be in a heightened state of arousal. Remember your ancient self in prehistoric times, back when your ANS and your environment were perfectly suited for each other? In those times, you wouldn't start mouth breathing unless you were in danger, on the hunt, or running from predators. When you mouth breathe, even when you are sitting on the couch watching TV, you are sending a signal to your ANS that you are being chased by a predator, that you are not safe, that you need to shut down your digestion and other systems that

are not vital to surviving a run-in with a lion or tiger. Subsequently, your body responds by making stress hormones. By simply mouth breathing, you have created a stressed state.

2. **A low CO2 tolerance.** This means that you will feel the hunger for air more quickly. You'll be out of breath at the top of the stairs, even though you run 5K every day. Simply put, you've become accustomed to a low level of CO2 because mouth breathing rids your system of CO2 much faster than nasal breathing. For athletes, switching from mouth breathing to nasal breathing is a game-changer because, in time, they are able to tolerate a higher level of CO2 in their blood, meaning they are capable of performing more intensely for longer periods of time without becoming "gassed," or unable to breathe fast enough to continue.

3. **Reduced immune effectiveness.** Let's not forget that the air that you inhale through your mouth is unfiltered and unaltered. It is not humidified or temperature controlled by the nasal passages. It is a raw product. Anything that is in the air when it enters through your mouth can make it all the way to the bottom of your lungs without being impeded by the natural filtration system in your nose.

Many people mouth breathe and don't even know it. I was one of those people. As a teacher and lecturer, I am constantly speaking. Without realizing it, I would be mouth-breathing all day long. Try to think about your breathing throughout the day. Are you mouth breathing or nasal breathing?

Tape Your Mouth Shut?

One most common instance of mouth breathing is during sleep. Imagine waking up after a full night's sleep and not feeling fully rested. Does that sound familiar? It might be that you are mouth breathing while you sleep, sending "fight or flight" signals to your autonomic nervous system, even though all you want is get some rest. This is more common than people realize. How do you solve this problem? Within the breathwork world, many people have resorted to taping their mouths shut to prevent unconscious mouth breathing during sleep. As strange as it might sound, this practice has been a life-changer for many people who had been living with chronic anxiety and sleep problems. I know it might sound a little excessive, but give it a try. You might thank me in the morning. My wife was a chronic mouth breather in her sleep, and when she began taping her mouth, she woke up feeling rested and experienced less stress throughout the day. This was literally an overnight change in her life, and it was all thanks to simply taping her mouth shut. (Yes, I suggested to my wife that she should tape her mouth shut, and yes, she actually thanked me.)

Chapter 15.

Inhales, Exhales, Apneas and How These Things Influence Your Autonomic Nervous System

When we think about yoga, martial arts, or any athletic pursuit, we generally break the activities down into separate parts. In yoga, there are separate positions that, when combined together, make an asana, or a sequence. In Brazilian Jiu-Jitsu, practitioners learn a variety of locks and holds to submit their opponents. In sports, there are different maneuvers or plays that can be combined into an offensive or a defensive strategy. These smaller parts of the activity can be combined in a nearly infinite number of ways to produce a session of yoga, rolling, sparring, or a game. Breathwork is no different. Once you understand the pieces, you can more fully understand the whole of a session or a technique.

Inhalation / Inspiration

Inhaling is an obvious component of breathing. In our breath-work practices, we can use inhales to signal a sympathetic state of arousal. This is quite evident when it is experienced from a "bottom up" experience, like being surprised or frightened—we gasp. When we use inspiration in our breathwork practice, we should be aware that it is a sympathetic signal.

Exhalation/ Expiration

Like every inhale, every exhale can be done in a variety of ways that we will discuss. In our breathwork sessions, we can use exhales to signal a parasympathetic state. This is also quite evident when we exhale from an event in our lives. We sigh when we are relaxed, satisfied, or relieved. These are natural and automatic aspects of exhalation that anyone can observe.

Apneas/ Kumbhakas/ Breath Holds

A breath hold is a powerful signal to the ANS, and it also allows for gas transfer to occur without respiration to assist in the elimination of carbon dioxide or the replenishment of oxygen. Breath holds are used for various reasons. Here are three breath holds commonly found in breathing techniques.

1. Full Lung/ Antara Kumbhaka- A breath hold with a full lung can be a sympathetic trigger, signaling an active and aroused state for most people. A long breath hold with a full lung will also allow for a long gas exchange, creating a longer breath hold than empty lungs. This can be useful for a variety of reasons that we will explore later.

2. Neutral Lung/ Kevala Kumbhaka- In this technique, the practitioner exhales air without forcing all of it out with the diaphragm. A neutral lung is generally a parasympathetic

trigger, sending a signal to the ANS to rest and relax the body. It should feel like a state of complete relaxation. No tension; the absence of doing anything.

3. Empty Lung/ Bahya Kumbhaka- Truly emptying the lungs is rarely used, since it can be uncomfortable. During an empty lung hold, the gas exchange will generally affect the practitioner earlier than in the previous two holds. This means that it's hard to hold for very long.

It is important to practice interoception when experimenting with apneas. While many people experience them the same way, many practitioners have told me that they feel an opposite reaction. For instance, while most practitioners will feel energized from breathwork involving a full lung apnea, some become more relaxed and parasympathetic. Again, you have to learn to listen to your own "inner voice" to best understand how these techniques affect you.

Chapter 16.

CO2 | The Need to Breathe

It is essential to understand the pulmonary trigger that causes one to feel the urge to breathe, CO2. While oxygen is vital for human life, it is not a low level of oxygen that causes one to feel the need to breathe. The urge to breathe is caused by the body's chemoreceptors sensing a buildup of CO2.

A Very Simplified Account of Cellular Respiration

Cellular respiration, the process by which each cell's mitochondria create ATP (cellular energy). The process consists of the following:

1. The mitochondria consume glucose and O2 to produce ATP
2. One of the byproducts of this process is CO2

Again, this a super-simplified explanation of the process for the purposes of making this part of the book as short and to-the-point as possible.

When we detect an uncomfortable level of CO2, we feel the urge to breathe. This urge becomes stronger and stronger, eventually painful, until we take our next breath. However, while our O2 level may be dropping somewhat throughout, O2 saturation generally does not dip significantly. When we are physically active, our mitochondria produces more ATP, and therefore more CO2. This is why we feel the increased urge to breathe when we are physically active.

Why Is a Higher Tolerance to CO2 Beneficial? | The Bohr Effect

One's CO2 tolerance (the amount of CO2 one can tolerate before feeling the urge to breathe) can be increased or decreased over time. A higher level of CO2 in the blood causes the red blood cells to deliver more O2 to the tissues. It is a strange fact, but when CO2 levels are lower, red blood cells bind too strongly to O2 to deliver it to your tissues. This is due to a phenomenon known as the Bohr effect, discovered in 1904 by Christian Bohr, which describes the inverse relationship between oxygen's bonding affinity and the acidity and concentration of CO2. Simply put, when you have low CO2, your red blood cells will not as readily release the oxygen that they are carrying, depriving your tissues of oxygen. With a higher level of CO2, red blood cells more readily release O2 from the blood to the tissues, which, of course, is very important for the performance of those tissues.

This means that person with a high tolerance for CO2 is capable of performing physically demanding activities longer than someone who has a low tolerance. Therefore, it is in an athlete's best interest to do everything possible to increase their CO2 tolerance. This is done naturally when we engage in physically demanding activities; however, many athletes have such poor breathing habits that they still have a low CO2 tolerance. This can be addressed directly with breathwork, and some of the exercises in this book do just that.

But what about the rest of us? What if I'm not a track star? Why should I care about my CO2 tolerance? Great question. It is still important for you too. I don't care who you are. If you are a human, you should care about your CO2 tolerance.

A person with a low CO2 tolerance will take more breaths per minute than one who has a high CO2 tolerance. This both reinforces their low CO2 tolerance and is likely to put them into a state of "fight or flight." The ANS is always listening. If your breathing is not slow and restful, it must mean that you are not in a safe place. The faster we breathe, the more likely we are to send ourselves into a sympathetic state, with all of the things that come with it. Again, this is fine if you are really in a situation where you need those stress hormones to help you survive, but not at the office, not at the dinner table, not when you are trying to sleep.

Here are two ways to test your CO2 tolerance:

The Body Oxygen Level Test

The Body Oxygen Level Test, or BOLT, assesses your CO2 tolerance. It is described in the book *The Oxygen Advantage* by Patrick McKeown, and it goes like this:

[Note: This is not a test to see what your maximum breath hold time is. It is best to take this test when you are not caffeinated. It is best if not done right after a meal.]

1. Come to a rested and relaxed position and breathe normally. This can be seated or lying down. Get a stopwatch or keep

time with your phone. You will be timing a short pause in your breathing.

2. Take three normal breaths and at the end of your third breath, exhale to a neutral lung.

3. Hold until you feel the first real urge to breathe.

4. Go back into normal breathing. NOTE – Your breathing should be relaxed and unstressed when you go back into breathing after the breath hold. You should not be gasping for air or breathing any harder than you did before the breath hold.

The ideal BOLT score is 40 seconds. But don't feel down if your time was lower. It is simply a test of where you are at this moment. As you engage in breathwork, you can start setting goals for your BOLT test. (See the chapter on increasing your CO2 tolerance)

The CO2 Tolerance Exhale Test

Another way to test your CO2 tolerance is using the following test. It is currently used by the elite trainer, Brian Mackenzie, and it is becoming more popular than the BOLT test. I prefer it to the BOLT test because I believe it is harder to cheat or mess it up. You will need a stopwatch to complete it. All breathing must be done through the nose. Here is how it is done:

1. In a comfortable position take three normal breaths.

2. Take one more breath, but this time, fill the lungs completely.

3. Start your stopwatch and start to exhale. Exhale as slowly as you can for as long as you can.

4. When you have no air left in your lungs or you are simply unable to continue the exhale, stop your timer. If you swallow,

stop your clock. If you hold your breath for any amount of time, stop the clock. You must use one slow continuous breath without any stops.

Basic meanings of scores:

Greater than 80 seconds: Elite. You have a high tolerance to CO_2 and you are skilled under stress.

Between 60 and 80 seconds: Advanced. Still very good. You have a healthy pulmonary system and great skill under stress. But guess what? You can probably improve even more.

Between 40 to 60 seconds: Intermediate.

Between 20 and 40 seconds: Average.

Lower than 20 seconds: Poor tolerance to CO_2 and probably in a high state of stress or arousal.

We experience CO_2 as a stressor. When we train our CO_2 tolerance, we are not only improving our CO_2 tolerance with time, we are training ourselves to be more resilient to stress. For more on CO_2 training, see Chapter 22.

BREATHING PROTOCOLS

Now that you have a better understanding of your breathing and how breathing works, let's dive into breathing techniques. The following breathing techniques will serve as a toolbox for you in your breathwork practice. As I said earlier in this guide, this is not an exhaustive list of all of the techniques and protocols that exist. This is a collection of breathing techniques that I use in my own practice, that I have tested on myself and others, and that are also in use by countless breathworkers and breathing specialists around the world.

Use the information we've explored up until now to enrich your breathing practice. Which protocols are associated with becoming more active and alert? Do they have short or long inhalations vs. exhalations? What do these protocols have in common? Where do you notice the biggest differences? Most of the techniques described in this guide are fundamentally based on what we know about how breathing affects our autonomic nervous system from the top-down.

Later in this guide, I will offer some guidance to create your own breathwork protocols. Perhaps you like one of the protocols I describe below, but in your own experience, you find that a small change is beneficial. This is fine. Breathwork is your birthright. You don't need anyone's permission to make changes if they produce a more desirable effect. However, before making changes or inventing your own, I encourage you to practice the protocols as they are described. These protocols have been tested by time and countless practitioners who have come before you. Benefit from their experimentation.

Chapter 17.

Breathwork Notation | The Four Corners of Breath

Most of the techniques described in this guide are described using what many breathing specialists call "the four corners of breath." This concept is illustrated below:

Full-Lung Apnea

Inhale   Exhale

Apnea After Exhalation

Using the four corners of breath, one can describe a breathing technique by how many counts/seconds a practitioner should spend on each of the four corners. For instance, a practice might be: inhale of four seconds, a full-lung apnea of four seconds, an exhale of four seconds, and an apnea after exhalation for four seconds. In notation, 4,4,4,4.

If we want to make the inhale and exhale longer—let's say 6 counts/seconds—the notation would be 6,4,6,4. If a number is 0, it means to skip that corner and go to the next one. For instance, if the notation is 4,0,4,4, you would inhale for four seconds, exhale for four seconds, and apnea with a neutral lung for four seconds; skipping any apnea with a full lung.

The order is always the same: Inhale, Full Lung Apnea, Exhale, Apnea After Exhalation.

Autonomic Nervous System Protocols

Reminder: Influencing the autonomic nervous system is not simply a matter of counting your breathing. It requires greater focus. All breathwork requires focus. You are trying to influence systems that should not be accessible, but they are. When you practice breathwork, this level of focus may not be easy at first. There is a real meditative quality to breathwork. With time and conscious efforts to improve your focus, it is possible to use your breath as a tool to make serious changes in your health and wellbeing. Just remember that it is a practice, not a magic spell. Your dedication to focus is crucial. This means clearing your mind of any thoughts other than the task you are performing while avoiding the tendency to become tense with hyper focus. Just stay relaxed with a clear mind. Observe your inner state and avoid judgmental thoughts that might cause you anxiety. I know all of this is easier said than done. That is why we practice.

Chapter 18.
Breathing Protocols to Calm Down

To encourage a parasympathetic state ("rest and digest"), you can enhance all of the following breathing techniques below by laying down, closing your eyes, relaxing your forehead, bringing a slight smile to your lips, and listening to soothing music. When lying down, bring your hips and knees to 90-degree angles, propping them on a chair or with your feet on the wall. These are all sympathetic triggers that can help you.

For every exercise in this section, breathe low into your belly, avoiding filling your chest. Your shoulders should not move with your breath. Ideally, your body is still, and your diaphragm is the only thing that moves. Avoid exaggerating the motions in order to get the tempos right. We are shooting for smooth, even, and controlled breaths.

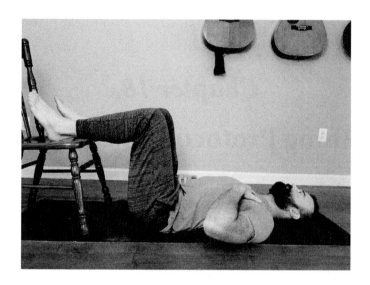

Bottom Triangle: Nasal Breathing Only (4,0,4,4) (5,0,5,5) (6,0,6,6) and so on…

For this breathing technique, your inhale, exhale, and neutral lung apnea should all be even times. There is no hold with a full lung.

No Full Lung Apnea

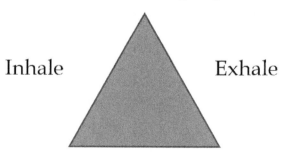

Inhale   Exhale

Apnea with Neutral Lung

1. In a comfortable position, find your natural breathing pattern. Before making any changes, observe where your breath is. This will help to inform your starting speed.

2. Begin your triangle with a tempo that is as close to your resting breath as possible; ideally, you will be able to find a 4,0,4,4 breathing tempo. Your inhales and exhales should be smooth and even. Your breath hold should be relaxing, without force or tension.

3. If you can complete this exercise easily for a period of a minute or two, try "growing your triangle" by extending your counts from 4,0,4,4 to 6,0,6,6. Likewise, if you find this to be easy to do for a minute or two, you can continue to grow your triangle as large as you like.

The most important thing to remember about any technique geared toward finding a parasympathetic state ("rest and digest") is that the breathing should be smooth and relaxed. If you feel like you are tensing up, or if you are experiencing heavy hunger for air during any part of this technique, throttle back to a smaller triangle with shorter periods of time for the inhale, exhale, and apnea.

If you strain or push yourself to discomfort, you will not send the appropriate signal to you ANS.

The 1:2 Breathing Ratio (4,0,8,0) for Vagal Stimulation

When we extend our exhale, we stimulate the vagus nerve and send a powerful signal to our ANS that we are in a calm and safe place. If I could teach you only one breathing technique, this would be it. It's incredibly simple, but that doesn't necessarily mean it's easy.

In a comfortable position, find your natural breathing pattern. Before you make any changes, observe where your breath is. This will help to inform your starting speed.

1. Making as little change as possible, bring your breathing pattern to a 1:2 ratio, Inhale (1) to Exhale (2). For every second you inhale, you will exhale for two.
2. Slowly, and without force, lengthen your inhales and exhales, keeping the ratio of 1:2.
3. Ideally you will find a 4:8 breathing pattern. You can keep this pattern as long as you like.
4. If you would like to go deeper into your parasympathetic state, continue to add time to your inhales and exhales.

Important Note: This technique only works if you stay relaxed in your body and smooth in your breathing.

The Anti Arousal Breathing Exercise

In their highly acclaimed book, *Recognizing and Treating Breathing Disorders: A Multidisciplinary Approach,* Leon Chaitow ND DO, Dinah Bradley DipPhys NZRP MNZSP, and Christopher Golbert PhD describe a simple breathing exercise that each of us can perform to reduce our state of arousal in a stressful state, bringing the practitioner a sense of calm. This technique is particularly powerful if you're feeling a bout of anxiety, fear, or overwhelm. (It is what Breathin' Steven should have done in Chapter 11.)

It goes like this:

1. In a seated or lying down position, inhale fully. Then slowly exhale all of the air from your lungs and use the "recoil" of your diaphragm to naturally provide you with an effortless inhale.

2. Exhale fully, and very slowly. In their instructions, they say to breathe a stream of air so gently that it would not blow out a candle if it were six inches in front of your mouth. The goal is to lengthen this exhale for as long as you can, counting each second as it passes. The goal is that your effortless inhales will be approximately two to three seconds while your exhales will be around six to seven seconds.

3. Repeat thirty breaths at this pace.

Balanced Breathing

This technique involves an even 1:1 ratio of inhales to exhales. There are no apneas; just smooth breath waves using nasal inhales. Exhales may use the nose or the mouth. In a seated or prone position, inhale for five seconds and exhale for five seconds. Continue this as long as possible, using smooth breaths.

A five-second inhale/exhale brings you to six breaths per minute, which stimulates your vagus nerve, eliciting a parasympathetic state. This effect can be increased by increasing your breath times as long as you can perform them smoothly. You may graduate to six seconds inhale/exhale, 10 seconds, etc.

Peaceful Apneas

One of the most relaxing things you can do with the breath is to take a deep inhale, let it go, and hold your breath with a neutral lung. This isn't a breath hold for any other purpose other than being completely relaxed. You are literally using none of your muscles at this point if you are lying down, not even your breathing muscles. The technique is simple

1. Take a deep breath in through your nose, and let it go.
2. Before breathing again, pause for just a few seconds and feel the peace of being completely at rest.

It's that simple. Try it any time you like.

Chapter 19.

Breathing Protocols to Activate

Activation breathing techniques are not for those who are pregnant or nursing. Check with your doctor if you are unsure if you are healthy enough for activation breathwork.

Top Triangle: Inhales are Nasal Only (4,4,4,0)

For this breathing technique, your inhale, full-lung apnea, and exhale should all be even times. There is no hold with an empty lung.

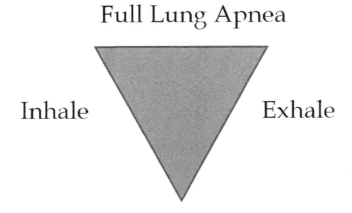

Full Lung Apnea

Inhale   Exhale

No Apnea with Neutral Lung

1. In a comfortable position, with a neutral spine, find your natural breathing pattern.
2. Take a deep breath all the way in, and let it go.
3. Come to a 4,4,4,0 breathing pattern, inhaling for four seconds, holding with a full lung for four seconds, then exhaling for four seconds.
4. Continue this pattern until you feel the desired effects.

Note: To intensify the effects of this technique, apply some light pressure to the breath hold and smile as you practice. This is one of my favorite ways to energize myself before workouts or when I just need a boost.

Pranayama Breathing Techniques for Activation

The following two breathing techniques come directly from the ancient Hindu Vedas. There are many claims attributed to these techniques, both spiritual and physical. Again, the focus of this book is simply the practical uses of breathing techniques. I will show respect to the traditional practice of pranayama by not trying to explain it in my own words. I leave that to yogi masters. My instructions and descriptions of their uses are simply from a secular point of view.

Kapalhbati (Skull Shining)

This is a yogic breathing technique that I have found useful for increasing energy. It strengthens your diaphragm and your accessory breathing muscles. I especially love this technique because it helps build neuromuscular control over your breathing muscles, and the focus required to practice this technique keeps one from wandering in thought, making it a meditative experience as well. In my experience, I find it quite energizing and pleasant.

This technique can also be a great primer for silent meditation, making it hard to simply lump it in with activation techniques. Try it for yourself and determine how it works for you—does it calm or energize? My primary reason for including it in the activation section is because it is a technique that I often recommend to athletes getting ready to train, and I often use it to activate my system before beginning other breathing techniques.

This technique can cause dizziness and disorientation when practiced. Do not practice this technique while driving or in water.

All breathing will be done using your belly. No chest breathing on this one. This technique consists of an active exhale with your abdominal muscles and diaphragm. The inhale is passive; you will passively allow air to re-enter your lungs via the recoil of your belly.

Control is what we are looking for. You might have seen this technique demonstrated in videos, and many practitioners can get very fast. Speed should only come with control. When you have mastered consistent, controlled breaths at a slow pace, you can increase your tempo. Faster is not better.

All breathing is done through the nose. You might want to have a handkerchief handy just in case mucus come out of your nose. Yes, it can get messy, but don't let that stop you! Later in this book, when we discuss how to put your own breathing sessions together, remember that this is a great technique for opening the nasal passages. This means that one can place it at the beginning of a session to improve all of the techniques that will follow.

1. Find a seated position. Lying down is also acceptable. The most important thing is that you have a neutral spine and are comfortable.
2. Push all the air out of your lungs using your abdominal muscles and allow your belly to recoil out. This will be your starting position.
3. Push out the air with your diaphragm and abdominal muscles with a single contraction. This will make a sharp exhale. Then allow your belly to relax. You should notice that you have taken in a small breath of air.
4. Repeat this process until you feel that you have energy; then take a deep breath, filling up the belly and the chest, and then exhale it out slowly.
5. Take some time to observe your body. What do you notice about your current state? Listen to your inner voice. Do you need another round? Are you satisfied with what you have done already? This is where you can practice interoception to guide you forward.
6. After you have finished your last set, you can take some time to meditate, or you can use your blissful state to propel you into your next activity.

Bhastrika (Bellows Breath)

Over the years, I have learned two distinct variations of Bhastrika, both from reputable teachers (remember when I said that experts disagree?). I practice both.

Technique 1:

This technique is very similar to Kapalhbati, but I recommend practicing Kapalhbati before learning Bhastrika. It offers many of the same benefits to Kapalhbati, but the active inhale and exhale requires a greater level of control over your abdominal muscles and diaphragm. This technique also usually involves a breath hold, which is how I recommend practicing it.

Again, all the breathing is through the nose. You might want to have a handkerchief handy just in case mucus comes out of your nose. Like Kapalhbati, when we discuss how to put your own breathing sessions together later, remember that this is a great technique for opening the nasal passages. This means that one can place it at the beginning of a session to improve all of the techniques that will follow. Like, Kapalhbati, this should be practiced in a safe location, because you might get light-headed.

1. Assume a seated position, arms open, hands resting palm-up on your legs or knee.
2. Push all the air out of your lungs using your abdominal muscles and allow your belly to recoil out. This will be your starting position.
3. Push out the air with your diaphragm and abdominal muscles with a single contraction; then inhale, using the same muscles, with a single contraction. The belly and ribs expand with each inhale and contract with each exhale. Each inhale and exhale should ideally be identical in size and strength. I imagine the sequence like a bellow working air in and out of your lungs.
4. Repeat this process, keeping a consistent cadence, with even inhales and exhales. Shoot for one breath per second in the

beginning, and approximately two breaths per second as you get the hang of it over time. Speed is not the primary goal, consistency is.

5. For beginners, repeat this process for 10 to 15 times. As you become more experienced in this technique, you can go longer, but in the beginning stick with short controlled rounds.

6. When you are ready, take a slow inhalation through the nose and fill your lungs completely, practicing a proper breath wave by pulling your breath down to your abdomen first and filling your chest last. Tilt your head back slightly as you complete your inhalation.

7. Once you have filled your lungs, tilt your chin down gently, forming an air lock in your throat. In pranayama this is known as Jalandhara Bandha, or the throat lock.

8. Hold your breath (Antara Kumbhaka) for as long as possible, without straining or forcing. When you feel the strong urge to breathe, slowly exhale through the nose. Bring your awareness within. Practice interoception. Observe the changes. This might also be a good time to meditate, taking advantage of the peaceful state you have created.

9. Take two or three relaxing breaths to recover, or even more if you feel the need. Once you are settled, you can go into another round.

10. Repeat as many times as you like. When you have finished, you can meditate or activate. The choice is yours.

Technique 2:

Again, all the breathing is through the nose. Eyes should be closed.

1. Come to a seated position.
2. Bring your hands next to the sides of your shoulders in a relaxed fist. Your elbows should be near your ribs.
3. Inhale as you raise your hands to the ceiling, opening them as you raise them.
4. Exhale, pulling your arms and hands back down to the starting position, bringing them to a relaxed fist.
5. Repeat steps 4 and 5 ten to fifteen times.
6. Bring you hands to your lap, palms up, and take a relaxing break. Observe the changes.
7. Repeat as many times as you like.

The motion resembles pushing an invisible bar up and then bringing it back down. You don't have to focus much on your breathing muscles when you practice this version of Bhastrika. Just allow the motion of your arms to do the work for you. Inhale normally as you bring your hands up as high as you can. Then allow your arms to drop as you exhale. The exhale will be much faster and with more force than the inhale. Don't worry about making this a fast thing. The usual speed is around one breath per 2 seconds.

Chapter 20.

Breathwork for "Stay and Play" | Flow State

Thus far, we've discussed the state of "fight or flight" and the state of "rest and digest," but what about a balanced state? Perhaps you are nervous about a situation where you will need to be sharp and ready to perform at a high level. You need to calm down, but you don't want to completely shut down. What do you do?

This is when breathwork can take us into a state of "stay and play." This is a balanced state that is ideal for finding "the zone," or what some people refer to as a "flow state." The following breathing techniques can be practiced a variety of ways, but I find that the following are the best methods for getting the most out of these techniques:

1. Inhales should be done through the nose only.
2. Exhales should be done through the mouth, but can be done through the nose without losing any effectiveness. Exhaling through the mouth provides a greater degree of control over your exhales.
3. Each breath should fill the entire lungs, so both belly and chest should be active.

4. Your ribs should flare out with every breath, but you should not lift your shoulders. Pay special attention to this.

5. During your full-lung apneas, smile.

Box Breathing

This technique is used by the US Navy SEAL teams to find their focus before missions. It involves even counts on all four sides of each breath, hence the name, "box breathing."

This can be done while moving around or driving, but be very careful. Practice this technique in a safe seated position first before practicing it in motion. To avoid dizziness that can sometimes come from the breath hold, don't pressurize the abdomen during the full-lung apnea.

Full-Lung Apnea

Inhale — Exhale

Apnea After Exhalation

1. In a comfortable position, find your natural breathing pattern. Before you make any changes, observe where your breath is. This will help to inform your starting speed.

2. Begin your "box" with a tempo that is as close to your natural breathing tempo as possible. Ideally you can begin with 4,4,4,4 or longer; however, if you are very aroused, you might be breathing faster than this. Don't worry about it. Just get into a smooth flow of inhale, hold, exhale, hold.

3. After you practice your starting tempo for two minutes, you can extend the sides of your "box." Again, 4,4,4,4 is generally ideal, so if you started with this, you can choose to stay there or lengthen as well.

   Your goal is to achieve a "flow state" or get into "the zone." This requires interoception. You need to be able to listen to the subtle language of your body and mind. This will mean that you have to listen closely to your state and use your intuition to guide you. For many, the ability to expand their "box" goes hand-in-hand with their ability to get into "the zone" or "flow state."

4. Practice this technique for as long as you need to achieve results. Remember that the more you practice this technique, the better you will be able to listen to the subtle changes within yourself and the better you will be able to find your desired level of focus.

4-7-8 Breathing | Cadence of Happiness

Full disclosure, the name "Cadence of Happiness" is my invention. Most breathworkers in the industry simply refer to this technique by the name "4-7-8 Breathing." I love this technique, but I use it for a different purpose than most breathworkers.

This technique is one that is commonly recommended for getting to sleep. While it is a relaxing technique, when practiced with a full lung as opposed to only filling the belly, I find this technique to be ideal for inducing a state of "stay and play." If you have ever seen me speak in public or on an interview, it is likely that I was practicing this breathing technique minutes before.

This technique can be practiced while moving around, but before you do that, practice it in a seated position, or lying down. Some people may feel dizzy on the full lung apnea, so just be careful when you practice it. To reduce the intensity of the dizziness, avoid pressurizing the lung (flexing the abdominal muscles) upon the full lung apnea. The time of each part of the breathing technique is not important; what is important is the ratio between each part, four counts for the inhale, seven counts for the full lung apnea, and eight counts for the exhale.

1. Inhale fully though your nose for four counts. Be sure to flare your ribs as you inhale.
2. Hold your breath with a full lung for seven counts. To intensify the experience, smile.
3. Exhale slowly through your mouth or nose for eight counts.
4. For beginners, just try four to eight rounds of this at first. Practice this technique as many times as you like each day. With regular practice, you may notice that you begin to feel like you are in a state of flow more often.
5. For more advanced practitioners, you can repeat this cadence for as long as you need. Pay attention to changes in your state.

4-1-8-0 Breathing | Competition Breathing

This technique is especially helpful right before a competition. You want to be alert and energized, but you don't want to be frantic or unfocused. It is easier than box breathing since it does not focus on breath holds as much, and it can be a great technique to use as you are walking out to the fighting ring, the podium, the interview, or the dance floor.

1. Inhale fully though your nose for four counts. Be sure to flare your ribs as you inhale.

2. Hold your breath with a full lung for one count. To intensify the experience, smile and lightly pressurize your abdomen.

3. Exhale slowly through your mouth or nose for eight counts.

4. You may repeat this as long as you like.

Kasper van der Meulen's "One Breath Break"

Breathworker, biohacker, and author of *Mindlift: Mental Fitness for the Modern World*, Kasper van der Meulen invented a really useful technique to down-regulate your nervous system and allow you to get a handle on your focus. I love it because it can be used without anyone knowing you are doing it. It is short, simple, and it works. I classify this technique as one that is perfect for creating a state of flow. It calms the nervous system enough to keep you from losing focus, but it doesn't put you to sleep! It can be practiced anywhere, anytime. I recommend trying it in different situations to see how it best suits you.

1. Take a full breath in through your nose, filling your lungs completely.

2. Hold your breath with a full lung for 2 – 5 seconds.
3. Exhale a relaxed breath out and hold your breath with a neutral lung.
4. Hold your breath with a neutral lung until you feel the need to breathe.
5. Inhale through your nose.
6. Repeat as needed, then return to normal breathing.

Chapter 21.

Breathing Protocols for Athletic Training Enhancement (Not Just for Athletes!!)

Before I get into this section, I want to say that these techniques are not only reserved for athletes. Being able to influence your autonomic nervous system is a skill that will benefit anyone with a body and a mind.

When I title this section around athletic training, I am saying that these techniques are especially useful for those who push their respiratory systems to full throttle. If you belong to this category, you need to be able to get into "the zone," activate your system, and to shift into "rest and digest" as quickly as possible after your performance so you can get the most out of your recovery time. This means that you will also use a lot of the techniques we already covered. However, there are some new things to think about, especially when considering applying breathwork to athletic performance.

I want you to think back to a competition or a training session where you gave 100%. As we say in the USA, "You didn't have anything left in your tank." (We love to use car references in the USA.) Can you think of a time like this?

Take a minute to remember the way that felt. Your breathing was likely incredibly active, but you still couldn't catch your breath. Maybe your lungs were burning, your stomach turning, your muscles screaming, your body too weak to do one more step, one more rep, one more motion. You might have been lying on the ground panting, covered in sweat.

What has to happen to get you to this point? A few things. Depending on your activity, you were likely able to handle the first minutes, or even hours, while staying in the aerobic zone. In other words, there was a time when your breathing was able to meet the demands put on it by your body. Your blood glucose and the oxygen that you consumed through respiration were able to produce enough ATP (cellular energy) to keep up with the demand.

But then what happened? You kept pushing. You crossed over your aerobic threshold and became anaerobic, which means your cells were starved for oxygen. This can happen faster or slower depending on the activity, but once this threshold is crossed, the amount of time you have until complete exhaustion is limited. This is normal, and it is a natural process.

But what if I were to tell you that you can extend your aerobic zone? What if I told you that you can improve your respiratory system so that the moment of complete exhaustion that you felt in that competition or training session happens seconds, or even minutes, later? Would that have made a difference in your performance? Would that extra few seconds or minutes of energy make a difference in how well you place in any given competition?

In addition to improving your posture and your breath wave, the keys to using breathwork to improve athletic performance is in the following:

1. Increasing your tolerance to CO_2
2. Improving your O_2 carrying capacity
3. Strengthening your diaphragm and increasing neuromuscular control.

Chapter 22.

Fixing Over-Breathing and Raising CO2 Tolerance

I recommend testing your CO2 tolerance before attempting to improve your CO2 tolerance so you have a measurable way to gauge your progress.

I also recommend working with a breath coach if you are an athlete seeking personalized routines to improve your CO2 tolerance.

Conscious Reteaching | Two Strategies

The easiest way to fix over-breathing is to eliminate common over-breathing habits such as mouth breathing, a dysfunctional breath wave, and poor posture. The breathwork exercises already discussed in this guide address these issues head-on, so implementing a regular breathing practice is vital. You had to learn to be an over-breather, so you have to unlearn too. This means that you need to make a conscious effort to retrain your breathing and check in with your breathing all throughout the day.

Here are two tips to keep you on track.

1. Set timers on your phone. Think this through before you set your timers. What are times of day that you are likely to have

dysfunctional breathing? When do you need a reminder to check in on your posture, your mouth-breathing, or your breath wave? Try to set reminders for times when you will actually be able to take time to do a self-check, but don't ignore times when you are working or when you are active. These are probably the times when you need a reminder the most.

2. Maintain a regular breathwork schedule. This is something that I will explore in detail later, but learning to dedicate at least 10 minutes three times per day is ideal. My recommended times are first thing in the morning, before eating lunch, and before bed. The idea is to reset your breathing so regularly that you will train yourself to breathe well all day (and night) long.

CO2 Tolerance Building Exercises | A Warning and a Promise

Not only can you reset your CO2 tolerance to "normal" levels, you can increase your tolerance to CO2. This means that you will be less exasperated when you tax your lungs, and your breathing pattern should be less likely to get out of control.

Here is the rub. CO2 is naturally uncomfortable to tolerate. Aversion to CO2 is one of the most primal aversions in nature. Even gnats and fruit flies have an aversion to CO2. So, while you train yourself to tolerate higher levels of this blood gas, it will not likely be a blissful experience. However, after training you will have a higher tolerance to CO2, and having a higher CO2 tolerance is quite blissful because you will be less exasperated and more relaxed all throughout the day.

The promise that I have for you is that, while it might feel uncomfortable at times, it is not harmful. You won't be in danger. I compare the discomfort of raising CO2 tolerance to the discomfort one feels when beginning exercise. It doesn't feel great at first, and everything in your being is crying out for it to stop. But when practiced methodically, exercise leads to a healthier and stronger body. The same thing happens when training your CO2 tolerance.

CO2 tolerance training allows you to keep your breathing relaxed and controlled for longer periods of time, extending your aerobic zone and delaying the onset of the anaerobic zone. It also means that when you get to the anaerobic zone, the feeling of being out of breath will also be delayed.

Big Bottom Triangle Technique
(Instructions for Bottom Triangle Above)

The Bottom Triangle technique is an athlete's best friend. Not only is it a strong parasympathetic ("rest and digest") signaling technique (for most people), it can be used as a tool for improving your CO2 tolerance. The goal is to practice this technique three times per day and shoot for extending the apnea.

NOTE – The goal of practicing this technique is to extend the apnea without getting tense or out of breath. This takes focus and control, so if you have trouble doing this, just practice Bottom Triangle. With time, you will be ready to lengthen your apnea. Have a look at the instructions below.

No Full Lung Apnea

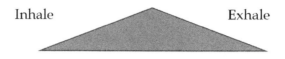

Inhale   Exhale

Apnea with Neutral Lung

1. In a comfortable position, find your natural breathing pattern. Before you make any changes, observe where your breath is. This will help to inform your starting speed.

2. Begin the Bottom Triangle Breathing Technique with a tempo that is as close to your resting breath as possible; ideally, you will be able to find a 4,0,4,4 breathing tempo. Your inhales and exhales should be smooth and even. Your breath hold between breaths should be relaxing, without force or tension.

3. Rather than lengthening your inhales and exhales, try to edge your apneas a little longer. Start very slowly and remain relaxed. For instance, perhaps you will go from 4,0,4,4 to 4,0,4,6. Stay with this new tempo for as long as possible while staying relaxed. If you find 4,0,6,4 to be easy, then you can extend the apnea even longer.

4. Practice this for ten minutes, three times per day. You can also do long sessions if you like.

The important thing to remember is that you are learning to tolerate CO_2 with this exercise. With each apnea, you are allowing the CO_2 to build up and test your comfort level. The key to lengthening your apnea is to relax. Don't try to fight it. You will never win this fight. Your goal is something more like falling in love with it. This is your body. This is CO_2 that you produced creating cellular energy to fuel your body. It isn't poison. It isn't harmful. Make friends with it. Fall in love with it. Reframe the sensation. No longer is it something that controls you. Now it is something that you can control.

Advanced Big Bottom Triangle Variables

When you have mastered Bottom Triangle, you can move to Big Bottom Triangle. When you have mastered Big Bottom Triangle, you can move to Advanced Big Bottom Triangle. Don't try to skip ahead in this progression. It is important to have trained yourself in the basics before adding variables.

Variation 1 | Bottom Triangle Breath Walking

Once you have had some luck with seated Big Bottom Triangle, you can practice Bottom Triangle Breath while walking. You may want to use your steps to keep time, or you can use a metronome, or simply count in your head if you are good at that. The goal is to keep the breathing pattern while walking. If you have to breathe through your mouth, shorten your triangle lengths or slow your walking.

I suggest doing this alone and without distraction.

Variation 2 | Bottom Triangle Stationary Bike

The goal of this exercise is to maintain the Bottom Triangle breathing pattern while riding a stationary bike. Keep your breathing smooth and as relaxed as possible. Find a speed on the bike that is comfortable and maintain that speed and breathing pattern for as long as you can. If you can keep the pattern and pace for five minutes, try speeding your peddling or lengthening the sides of your triangle.

Again, try to practice this in a place where you are not distracted.

Variation 3 | Bottom Triangle on a Row Machine

The goal of this exercise is to maintain the Bottom Triangle breathing pattern while rowing. Keep your breathing smooth and as relaxed as possible. Find a speed on the rower that is comfortable, and maintain that speed and breathing pattern for as long as you can. If you can keep the pattern and pace for five minutes, try speeding your rowing or lengthening the sides of your triangle.

Remember Rule #1 – Breath training is focus training. Learn to focus without force. To find ease in your breathing pattern while finding ease in your exercises.

Advanced Balanced Breathing

This technique involves an even 1:1 ratio of inhales to exhales. There are no apneas; just smooth breath waves using nasal inhales. **Each count must be one second.** Exhales may be through the nose or the mouth.

This technique can also be paired with exercise to improve CO_2 tolerance and cut down on suffering from an adrenaline dump that will leave you gassed.

Variation 1 | Balanced Walking

Walk as quickly as you can while maintaining a 5,0,5,0 breathing tempo. You may want to use your steps to keep time, or you can use a metronome, or simply count in your head if you are good at that. The goal is to keep the breathing pattern while walking. Try to find a speed that challenges you to keep this breathing pattern but one that you are able to maintain. If you can't keep the pattern, slow your walking pace.

Variation 2 | Balanced Stationary Bike

The goal of this exercise is to maintain the 5,0,5,0 breathing pattern while riding a stationary bike. Keep your breathing smooth and as relaxed as possible. Find a speed on the bike that is comfortable and maintain that speed and breathing pattern for as long as you can. If you can keep the pattern and pace for five minutes, try speeding your peddling or lengthening your breaths.

Variation 3 | Balanced Row Machine

The goal of this exercise is to maintain the 5,0,5,0 breathing pattern while rowing. Keep your breathing smooth and as relaxed as possible. Find a speed on the rower that is comfortable and maintain that speed and breathing pattern for as long as you can. If you can keep the pattern and pace for five minutes, try speeding your rowing or lengthening your breaths.

One Last Note on Combining Breathing Techniques with Exercise...

Of course, you can apply these breathing techniques to other forms of exercise. Start with simple movements and work your way up to more complex movements. Remember that training your breathing with simple motions like walking and stationary biking will help to build the mind/body connection that you need when trying more complex physical movements. You are consciously controlling your breath, which is normally automatic, during activity that requires your conscious control. Give yourself time to adapt.

The Added Bonus of Practicing the Techniques Mentioned Above...

Not only will the above techniques improve your CO_2 tolerance when practiced faithfully, they will extend your time in a parasympathetic state. Remember that you are using nasal breathing, and the techniques in this section keep you breathing at a slow and controlled pace. This prevents you from crossing over into "fight or flight" for longer, and with time, you will be able to be very active without being in a "fight or flight" state.

What are the implications of staying in a parasympathetic state for longer? Have you ever seen a martial arts pro who is so skilled that s/he defeats an opponent without any show of effort? Some of them are so skilled that they almost seem half-asleep while their opponents huff and puff and strain every muscle.

What you are seeing is two people who are in different states. When we are in a state of "fight or flight," the heightened levels of adrenaline (epinephrine) and noradrenaline (norepinephrine) can cause us to move frantically, releasing too much energy and making us lose control. With practice and skill, a trained martial artist knows that s/he does not need to use so much force, that the mind is one's greatest tool in any confrontation. Countless hours of practice have taught the skilled martial artist to stay calm rather than succumb to panicked movements. This provides a mental edge and saves valuable energy.

When we practice controlled breathing during exercise, we teach ourselves to stay calm when we are in an active state.

Chapter 23.

Hypoxic Training

Hypoxia is the state of low oxygen saturation in the body, generally anything lower than a blood oxygen saturation of 95%. It is usually a bad thing. However, when experienced in short doses in safe conditions, one can train their respiratory system to be stronger, increasing red blood cell count and allowing for greater oxygen transport capacity. But how can we bring our blood oxygen levels down safely?

Many people train in high elevations to get the benefits of low oxygen training, but athletes who understand and practice breathwork do not have to. Achieving a low blood oxygen saturation is quite easy with breathwork.

If you were to simply stop breathing, your mitochondria would continue to use oxygen in the process of cellular respiration. We discussed this process earlier in this guide. Since your blood is saturated with oxygen, even if you don't add any new oxygen to your blood for quite some time, the process of cellular respiration still continues, thanks to oxygen already in the blood. Of course, the longer you go without adding any new oxygen to your blood, the lower that saturation becomes, and eventually it will all be used up if you never take another breath.

But you can't help but take another breath. It is simply hard-wired through your autonomic nervous system to continue breathing. Even if you pass out due to low blood oxygen levels, your autonomic nervous system will turn your breathing back on while you are unconscious.

Of course, your body has a very effective safety measure in place to keep you from holding your breath to the point of passing out due to low oxygen levels. Breathing is triggered by CO_2, and no matter how great your tolerance is to CO_2, you will eventually be unable to resist the urge. You will take another breath.

But what happens when we delay the urge to breathe by exhaling CO_2 in larger quantities than normal? This is the foundational principle of Hypoxia Training; we rid our bodies of CO_2 at a rate significantly lower than our natural CO_2 tolerance. Doing this delays the urge to breathe and allows us to burn off oxygen in the blood to levels far lower than 95%. This puts us in a brief state of hypoxia, creating a stimulus that encourages our respiratory system to adapt.

Hypoxia training has been shown to increase the hormone EPO, which leads to an increase in the number of red blood cells. Red blood cells are responsible for carrying oxygen throughout the body, a boost that athletes have experienced for decades. In 2019, the Nobel Prize in Medicine was awarded to William Kaelin, Jr., Peter Ratcliffe, and Gregg Semenza, who discovered the exact mechanism behind this process. I'm not going to go into it, but if you would like to know more about this process, you can check out some of the research through the sources at the end of this book.

How to Determine Your Blood Oxygen Saturation

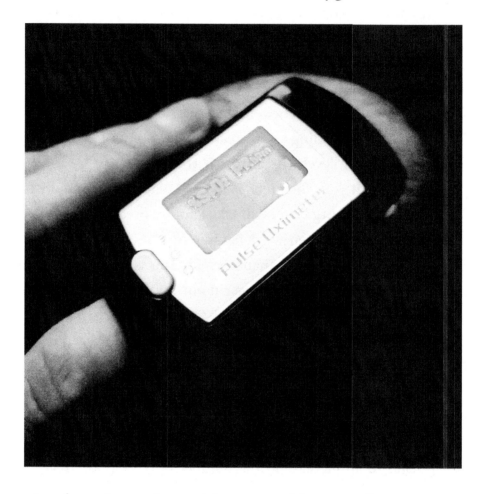

A pulse oximeter is a quick, easy, and low-cost device you can use to determine your blood oxygen saturation. You probably recognize this device from doctor visits. In normal situations, your reading should be between 95% and 100%, listed on the %SpO2 side. As you can see in the picture above, one can bring this number down significantly by practicing hypoxic breathwork. If you intend to get the full benefits of hypoxic training, I recommend picking one of these up.

SAFETY WARNING BEFORE PERFORMING HYPOXIC TRAINING

These protocols are not for those who are pregnant or nursing. If you suffer from epilepsy or uncontrolled high blood pressure, do not practice these techniques.

Please note that when one practices any breathing technique that causes a low blood oxygen saturation, it is essential to practice in a seated or lying down position ON THE FLOOR! Never practice these techniques near water or while driving. You will likely feel very dizzy, and it is possible to pass out. You may feel tingling, you might even feel some muscles tense up. These are all normal when practicing the following protocols. Only practice these techniques in an environment that is safe, free of sharp edges or other hazards that you might bump your head on if you suddenly fall unconscious.

If you do pass out, the only real risk is mechanical injuries caused from falling down. As I said earlier, no matter how long you hold your breath when conscious, if you become unconscious, your autonomic nervous system will restart your breathing process automatically. Your O2 levels will normalize very quickly, and you will return to your natural state. Always take these precautions seriously.

We will discuss the euphoric feeling that you get when practicing this kind of breathing technique in a later section. For now, let's be clear. Yes, it will feel good, but it should never be done outside of a safe environment. (I hope I beat this into the ground enough to make it clear that it is important!!)

Hypoxia Training Protocols

Standard Super Ventilation Technique

To take advantage of a delayed CO_2 trigger, all you need to do is blow off excessive amounts of CO_2. This can be achieved as easily as the following process:

1. In a safe place, using a neutral spine, take 15 to 30 deep breaths using a 1,0,1,0 tempo.
    a. Note: Breathe through your nose or the mouth, and use a full breath wave with each breath. Inhales and exhales will be active.
2. After your last deep breath, exhale to a neutral lung and hold your breath until you feel the strong urge to breath.
3. Repeat this process between three to four times, then return to normal breathing.

The Wim Hof Method Breathing Technique

Wim Hof's breathing technique also puts a practitioner in a brief state of hypoxia. I highly recommend learning it, and if you want to learn it well, I recommend finding one of my fellow instructors to teach it to you so that you can practice the complete Wim Hof Method. If you cannot learn it from an instructor, there are resources on his website to guide you, including a free mini-class that contains a video of Hof instructing you through the basics of the breathing technique. You can check it out today. I will warn you, you might also fall in love with cold showers!

To learn the complete Wim Hof Method visit: www.WimHofMethod.com

The Extreme Hypoxia Super Ventilation Technique (2:2 with sips)

This is the tool that I use most often with my athlete clients. From my own experience and the experience of the practitioners I have trained, this technique will result in the lowest O2 levels safely possible.

1. At a tempo of 2,0,2,0 take deep inhales and exhales, using a proper breath wave. You should inhale through the nose if possible and exhale through the mouth.
   a. Your inhalations should be full breath waves; belly, flared ribs, full chest. Your exhalations should be controlled, using the proper breath wave for exhalation.
   b. Exhales should not completely empty the lung. They should return to a position of neutral lung.
2. Repeat this breathing tempo for two minutes.
3. After two minutes have passed, take one last deep breath in and relax the exhale to a neutral lung.
4. You will hold for two minutes.
5. Small Sips of Air - If you feel the strong urge to breathe, take a small sip of air through your nose and out of your mouth and return to the apnea. Keep these very small. Do this as many times as you need to make it to the end of the two-minute apnea.
6. Repeat this three to five times. [NOTE: In time, you may decide to lengthen your breath hold time to up to three to five minutes. Only do this if you can consistently hold your breath for the full two-minute apnea, for at least three times in a row.]

Why does this work best to achieve hypoxia? It is all in the sip. And taking the proper sip of air is key to making this technique work better than others for a state of hypoxia.

Ideally, when we take the sip of air, we are clearing the lung of CO_2 without significantly oxygenating our blood. This requires practice, and you will need to monitor your results with your Pulse Oximeter to really know if you are doing it right. While we can sense high levels of CO_2, it is nearly impossible for us to sense low O_2 (which is why the Pulse Oximeter was invented in the first place). Let your breath sips be small and subtle. Just enough to release some CO_2, nothing more.

A Note on Breath Hold Times

One of the most common questions that I get when training people in hypoxic breathing techniques is about the apnea times. What normally happens is that the hold times are out of this world early on, and then after three to nine months, people notice that their breath holds level off (they stop seeing gains in apnea times) or they even reduce.

Lots of people worry about this. This is why I do not recommend timing the apneas. It doesn't help you. The thing to measure is your O_2 saturation. Are you consistently bringing your O_2 levels down with every session? This is the goal, not to hold your breath for long periods of time. Yes, the longer you hold your breath, the lower your O_2 saturation will generally drop. However, this is all dependent on how quickly your mitochondria are producing CO_2 and how high your CO_2 tolerance is. Other factors such as stress, what you ate in the past 24 hours, how much sleep you got the night before, etc. can also affect your apnea times. Some of these things can be helped, and some of them cannot. Do not get too wrapped up in the times.

However, if you are interested in lengthening your apnea times, you should also be practicing CO2 tolerance training.

A Note on Hypoxic Breathwork

Hypoxic breathwork is popular, and you will see lots of variations of what I have described above. It is important to understand the underlying principle upon which this style of breathwork is built. You are creating an imbalance in your blood gasses that pressures the body into becoming stronger and more capable. Changes in performance can take time, so don't expect anything overnight. However, with time and regular practice, a practitioner can see incredible benefits.

There are also other things happening in your brain when you practice super ventilation techniques like the ones described in this chapter. Learn more about what happens in your brain when you practice these techniques in Chapter 26.

Chapter 24.

Pre and Post Exercise

Breathing Protocols

When we workout, we should be mindful of our breathing, but let's face it, you also have a lot of other things to focus on. Perhaps you are playing a sport or doing some other activity that demands a lot of your attention. It is during these times that we are fortunate that breathing is also automatic. However, before each workout, we can set ourselves up for success by spending just a few minutes in conscious breathing.

Pre-Exercise Protocols

The Jolly Green Giant

This breathing exercise gets its name from the position in which you will stand. I also recommend smiling and finishing with a few laughs, but that is just me. The goal of this exercise is to activate your system and encourage a proper breathing pattern. Practice daily to fully internalize proper breathing.

1. In a standing position, place your hands on the middle of your ribcage.

2. Take a slow but deep breath in through your nose, using the proper breath wave (belly, ribs, chest). As you inhale, be sure that you feel your rib cage expanding as you pull your breath downward to your belly. Then fill your chest with air.
3. Exhale actively through the nose.
4. Repeat this at a slow pace for ten breaths.

5. Next, speed up the pace of your inhales and exhales, inhaling through the nose and out through the mouth. Continue to keep your hands on your mid-ribs and be sure they move with your rib expansion.
6. Repeat this for a minute.

7. Next, switch to mouth breathing for your inhales and exhales, making sure to use the proper breath wave and rib expansion.
8. Repeat this for a minute.
9. When you are finished, you can start your workout with the confidence that you have set your breathing pattern up for success.

Using Your Toolbox…

Many athletes ask if there are other things that should or could be done to improve exercise performance. This is where you need to look into your toolbox and decide for yourself. What do you need?

I'm tired from a long day at work… In this case, if you are still a little sluggish after doing your Jolly Green Giant routine, check the chapter on breathing protocols to activate the system. Maybe you should do some Top Triangle. Or, perhaps you should try Kapalbhati. Breathwork is your war chest, and will help you become a warrior in the gym!

Perhaps you are too amped up! Maybe you are stressed, or nervous. No problem. Check the chapter on protocols that can be used to induce a flow state, the "stay and play" state. Perhaps you should do a few minutes of Box Breathing to balance your ANS. Did that not work? No problem, either repeat the protocol for a longer period of time, or choose a different tool from your toolbox.

Wherever you are physically and mentally, you can apply a breathing protocol to improve your state and put yourself into the best position for a great workout or competition.

When the Workout is Over…

A sympathetic state is useful during exercise. It activates the skeletal muscle and prepares the body for action; however, once you have completed your workout, the ideal state for recovery is a parasympathetic state. Before you leave the gym, the track, the studio, etc. it is beneficial to take a few minutes to "downshift" your state in order to facilitate the most effective use of your out-of-the-gym time.

To accomplish this goal, return to the section about breathwork for a calm system and choose a technique that works best for you. Before you eat your post-workout meal, before you even leave the gym, find a quiet place and use one of the techniques described in the Breathwork for Calming Down chapter.

I recommend making this a habit that's penciled into every workout schedule. No matter if you are bodybuilding, playing a high impact sport, or simply playing a game of basketball with your friends, assume that you will spend 5 to 10 minutes shifting your ANS to a state of "rest and digest" before going home.

Chapter 25.

Breathing Exercises to Enhance Breathing Muscles Strength and Neuromuscular Control

One way that I try to make breathwork available for everyone is through the online application called Patreon. Each month I create a new guided breathwork session that members can enjoy. It's my way of bringing my breathwork sessions to places where I cannot be physically present. When Covid 19 began to hit the world, I had a lot of requests to focus on breathing exercises that would increase breathing strength. Even as I write this, the truth about Covid 19 is very unclear, but one thing that many who had contracted the virus had reported was difficulty breathing. So, we began to focus on exercises that focus on strengthening the diaphragm and the accessory muscles. These exercises are also great for athletes and anyone who wants to be a stronger breather.

Below are some exercises that improve breathing strength and neuromuscular control over the diaphragm. In Chapter 29, I provide a framework for how to put breathing exercises together to create a session. I have put two sessions specifically designed for increasing breathing strength and diaphragmatic neuromuscular control there for you. They are titled "Warrior Lung 1" and "Warrior Lung 2."

Ocean Breathing

This technique is named after the sound that this technique creates. The sound you will make when you are practicing this technique will resemble the long whooshing sound of waves crashing on the beach. This technique is also known as Ujjayi Breath by yogis and is commonly practiced in Ashtanga Vinyasa Yoga. This form of breathing can be done in any position, and it can be added to other timed breathing techniques to help the practitioner gain better control.

To practice this technique, you will need to close the back of your throat enough to slow breathing down. This is the same way you might slightly close the back of your throat to fog up a window or mirror. Holding some light tension in the back of your throat, with a closed mouth, breathe in and out of your nose slowly. It should be difficult to breathe fast because you are maintaining the gentle tension in your throat. At no time should this be uncomfortable or strenuous. Follow the directions below to get you started.

1. Take a deep breath, using the proper breath wave.
2. Gently close the back of your throat enough to provide resistance to your exhalation, just as described above, as if you are trying to fog up a mirror.
3. Exhale slowly. You should have to apply a little pressure to your exhalation to overcome the resistance in your throat. While you are exhaling, you should use the proper breath

wave, focusing on every bit of the wave, on the muscles you are using, and on the way this technique makes you feel.

4. Continue to exhale until you have exhaled approximately 90% of the air in your lungs.

5. Now inhale using the same resistance in your throat, focusing on every part of the breath wave as air enters your lungs. Fill your lungs as much as you can, using a complete breath wave. [However, if you would like to focus on lower breathing only, just do that. This technique is perfect for focusing on internalizing the breathing pattern that you choose.]

6. Repeat this process. You may choose to only do ten breaths, or you may choose to go for ten minutes. The most important thing is that you keep a consistent rate and evenly balance your inhales and exhales.

7. Again, it is important to remember that your breath should maintain a consistent rate. Speed is not important. If you feel uncomfortable, slow down your breath or speed it up to be comfortable, but keep each breath steady.

As you practice this technique, there should always be a little bit of tension between your effort to inhale/exhale and your throat.

What does this exercise accomplish? By slowing your breath down and providing resistance, you are forcing your nervous system to focus on what you are doing. You are allowing your breathing muscles to fully experience the breath wave with time enough to focus on every feeling and sensation that comes with it. You are slowing down a motion that we often perceive to be a single event, inhale or exhale, into a series of events that produce an inhale or a series of events that become an exhale. You are fully experiencing every station on that path, and as a result, with focus, you can learn to gain far more control over the muscles involved. Where you might have started this practice like a baby with a rattle, you can train your breathing muscles to have the precision of a surgeon with a scalpel.

In addition to those benefits, this technique can be very relaxing. Just think about why this might be. Remember, since we are slowing down our breathing, we are sending a "top down" signal to our ANS that we are safe. It is an excellent way to get into a resting state or to calm down from a "fight or flight" state. I have often found it helpful in calming my breath when I first get into an ice bath.

Reverse Straw Technique

This technique is fun and will make you a hit at parties. Well, maybe just parties where people like you and I like to attend. The reverse straw technique applies a resistance to your breathing muscles, providing a training stimulus to increase their strength. What makes this a funny technique to observe is that all of the resistance comes from your lips.

1. Exhale 70% to 90% of the air out of your lungs.
2. Purse your lips as if you are about to drink out of a straw.
3. Now, with strength, inhale through your pursed lips only, using the proper breath wave.
4. During your inhalation, you may slowly open your lips to allow for a reduction in resistance. This will vary depending on how you want to train. We will talk about this later.
5. At the end of your inhale, your mouth should be more open than at the beginning. Most of the time, your mouth will be

open as if you are saying "ahhh" after taking a big refreshing drink.

6. Relax all of your breathing muscles as you exhale. The exhale should be effortless and restful.

7. Repeat.

This exercise can be done in a variety of ways. I tend to describe them by describing the "length of the straw." The length of the straw refers to how long it takes to inhale the breath completely. This will vary depending on how long you keep your lips pursed in the starting position. In other words:

To make a "short straw": begin opening your mouth soon after the beginning of the inhalation. This will shorten the inhale. Your resting time between "straws" will only be the time it takes to take a relaxed exhale. When we practice short straws, we are practicing the Reverse Straw Technique with high repetitions.

To lengthen your straw: all you have to do is delay opening your lips. The longer the straw, the more your breathing muscles will experience time under tension; however, you will do fewer repetitions.

So, what is the ideal straw length? Well, it is like asking what is the ideal number of reps or sets or weight to lift. All of them are important, so try to practice this exercise with different lengths, and see what works best for you. You can see how I use this technique in the Warrior Lung sessions in Chapter 29.

Chapter 26.

Breathing for Meditation

Meditation is the easiest thing in the world. You just sit there and don't think of anything. Yes, I am still making jokes. What seems to be such a simple act is actually quite difficult for most of us. All of the data on meditation says that it is incredibly beneficial, yet most people who begin a meditation practice fail to keep it up. It is a shame too, because the majority of benefits of meditation come after regular practice over many years. The challenge people encounter is the flood of thoughts and anxieties that come when we stop our busy pace and sit in silence. That is when our inner chatter gets the best of us.

There are two very effective breathing practices that you can use to improve your meditation sessions. I'm sure there are many more, but I offer the following two so that you might have a starting place.

1:2 Ratio Breathing

A breathing ratio of 1 count per inhale for every 2 counts for an exhale is the ideal breathing pattern to stimulate your vagus nerve and come into a rested and relaxed state, one that will allow you to calm the mind and body. The slower, the better. This breathing should be done through the nose only, as long as you are able. Start with a 4,0,8,0 cadence, and if you can comfortably lengthen your breaths, do so. If you cannot lengthen your breaths comfortably, do not. The goal is to bring about a state of relaxation and calm so that you can clear your mind. If we get into an uncomfortable breathing pattern, we aren't going to create a meditative state. Just relax and find the best tempo for you.

Observing

Another method for improving your meditation is to simply observe yourself breathing. For many of us, and I'm included here, it is a difficult thing to simply observe yourself breathing. First of all, as you become aware of your breathing, you tend to take conscious control of it. But that is not the goal. When we simply observe our breath, we sit with ourselves, with our most intimate nature. Just observe and do not pass judgement. For many, this is a beautiful way to relax. For others, this may not be a great choice. It is all up to you.

Using a Prayer or Mantra

For millennia, humans have noticed that after a session of prayer or meditation using mantras, they feel calmer and more relaxed. This may very well be because of a spiritual connection made during this practice, but one thing that repeating a prayer or mantra will do for your breathing is set a pattern. All words have syllables, and syllables are the time-keepers in prayers and mantras. If you repeat a word, a sentence, or a paragraph over and over again, even silently, it is natural that you will change your breathing to accom-modate the syllables. If you don't like counting out time as you breathe, consider using a prayer or a mantra. Some people repeat sentences of empowerment or gratitude.

All of these things are great substitutes for counting. Whether you are religious, spiritual, or none of the above, it is worth giving this time-tested method of breathwork a try.

Chapter 27.

Superventilation as an Interrupter to the Dopamine Feedback Loop

Even with the assistance of the breathing techniques I described above, clearing our minds can be very difficult. The dopamine feedback loop can keep us from quieting our thoughts, and for many of us, the act of sitting down to meditate, eliminating all other forms of distraction, can seem to open the doors to more rumination. You might know what I am describing from your own experience; no longer do you have a list of outside distractions to keep you from thinking about regrets or the worries of the day. For many of us, when we attempt to meditate, we seem to invite rumination. The dopamine feedback loop strikes again!

We need an interrupter. Let me explain.

Have you ever had what seemed like would be an awful week, but then something different and unexpected happened that interrupted things and made you look at your week in a different way? Maybe you were in a state of despair and out of the blue, you bump into a friend you have not seen in a long time and shared some laughs. Or maybe you decided to try something new and exciting, like parachuting. You experienced an interrupter. Something that gave you a short break from the train of thoughts that you were stuck in, something that helped nudge you out of your malaise.

Superventilation is my preferred interrupter. But unlike many of the other things I have tried, superventilation is free and actually good for you. This can take the form of any of the breathing techniques covered in Chapter 23 on hypoxic training. Yes, these techniques have the capacity to improve our athletic performance, but superventilation is also a shortcut to a deep meditative state, a way to silence the chatter of the mind.

When we practice superventilation techniques like the ones described in Chapter 23, we are influencing our ANS with strong triggers, both sympathetic ("fight or flight") and parasympatetic ("rest and digest"). Just apply what you have learned about how breathing influences the ANS and think about why this is happening.

Let's suppose you are practicing the Extreme Hypoxia Superventilation Technique. Taking deep breaths at a fast pace (2,0,2,0) will send a strong sympatethic signal, activating your body and mind. Then we practice a neutral lung apnea. How does this affect our ANS?

Let's examine the long neutral lung apnea that follows, using what we know about how slow breathing affects the ANS. It doesn't get any slower than *not breathing*. Combined with the fact that we are using a neutral lung apnea and relaxing the body, we are sending a very strong parasympathetic signal to the ANS.

The strength of these signals is what makes this style of breathwork such a powerful interrupter. Changing your states with such extremes practically must interrupt the state that you were in when you first started the breathing session. So often, we are stuck in an emotional state, a chronic state of rumination or despair. Superventilation allows us to break out of that state.

Superventilation and Brain Activity

When we practice superventilation, something interesting occurs in our brains. As we exhale large amounts of CO_2, the result is a vasoconstriction in the brain that deprives the Neocortex of oxygen, briefly reducing activity in this area of the brain. The Neocortex is responsible for problem-solving, critical thinking, language, and rational thinking. When we practice superventilation, we briefly silence this part of our brain, escaping the chatter and creating a shortcut to deep meditation.

The end effect is a blissful, peaceful experience. In just a matter of minutes, we are able to do what only Olympic level meditators can do, silence our minds.

When we return to normal breathing, the brain normalizes in a matter of minutes. As bad as depriving your brain of oxygen sounds, it is harmless as long as it is done safely (see Chapter 23).

Emotional Breakthroughs as a Result of Practicing Superventilation

Many people have emotional responses when they practice superventilation techniques. This is normal, and those who experience these reactions generally either cry or laugh, arriving on the other side of the experience feeling as though they are better off.

I often feel a unique emotional state of the safety I once felt as a child when I was in the back seat of my parents car on our way home from church, looking forward to my mother's Sunday lunch. Yes, that emotional state is what I feel most commonly, and I am so thankful that I get to feel that emotional state again now, decades later. It is interesting that it took practicing breathwork to bring this emotional state out. I never would have thought about it on my own.

When I tell people about this, some people recoil. Many of us have very emotionally charged memories that we would like to avoid facing again. To this I must say two things.

1. Just because you avoid something does not mean that it isn't still hiding in your limbic system somewhere. It is likely coloring your every experience in life, meaning that you might be suffering from a memory or an emotional trauma, even after successfully "forgetting it" consciously.

2. I have guided countless numbers of practitioners through intense superventilation sessions, and everyone has reported a sense of leaving behind some kind of weight after the release. Sufferers of PTSD, abuse, and violence have reported feeling freer and "lighter" after regular practice of superventilation breathwork. Many report that they feel as though they were actually able to process the experience rather than run from it. And what is even greater, they say that they do not relive the event. Rather, they report being able to observe the emotion as if from a safe distance. They process the emotion, choosing to let it go or to keep it.

So often, in the West, we try to bury our emotions in rationality and practicality. Just look at me! I buried every emotion, anxiety, and discomfort in drugs. What superventilation does for us is provide a safe a non-addictive remedy for those of us who are stuck in our thoughts, our ruminations, our trauma.

Why exactly does it work? It is still not fully understood. After years of practicing and instructing this kind of breathwork, it is clear to me that, when practiced safely, superventilation is a great interrupter for the dopamine feedback loop. It quiets our worried minds, and briefly takes us into a state that allows us to process emotions and find peace.

I practice superventilation every day; sometimes I practice it many times in one day. If I notice that I am experiencing a high level of stress and anxiety, I try to make time to do more super-ventilation sessions. It is a tool that you have at your disposal to interrupt the mind's chatter when you need a break.

Tetany: Muscle Spasms/ Crab Hands/ Mantis Hands/ Involuntary Mudra

Many people experience muscle spasms or cramps in their hands, arms, toes, and even face when practicing superventilation breath-work. While there are many names attributed to the phenomenon, the scientific name for it is tetany. This condition can be caused by many things, but with regards to breathwork, it is caused when CO_2 levels drop in the blood, resulting in the kidneys produc-ing more bicarbonate, making the blood become more alkaline. I will spare you all of the details. The reason I bring it up is because people often wonder... *what is going on!?!?!*

Tetany, as a result of controlled superventilation (as described in Chapter 23), is harmless, and it will subside when you begin to breathe normally again. It is generally not an unpleasant experience for most practitioners, but if you begin to experience it, and you want it to stop, just go back into normal breathing or slow down your superventilation. Personally, I enjoy it when it happens to me.

What if I don't feel Tetany?
Am I doing something wrong?

Nope. Tetany is just something that occasionally happens. It isn't a measure of success or failure.

Chapter 28.

Altered State Breathing Techniques

WARNING – Altered state breathwork should not be practiced by women who are pregnant or nursing. If you suffer from epilepsy, do not practice altered state breathwork. If you suffer from any health condition, check with your doctor before attempting any form of altered state breathwork.

Like so much of breathwork, altered state breathwork is nothing new. Shamans and yogis discovered that using a combination of extended deep breathing, breath holds, and muscle squeezes, one can achieve a state that is normally impossible. Over the years, master breathworkers have adapted, rediscovered, and modified ancient techniques, but they usually all involve the same elements: a period of deep breathing where one increases energy, a breath hold, and some kind of muscle contraction. Not all altered state breathing techniques utilize all three of these elements, and many incorporate more steps, specific breathing patterns, bodywork, specific positions, and spiritual guidance. When it comes to altered state breathwork, there are many teachers, and there are many techniques. What is described in this chapter is what breathworker Kasper van der Meulen calls his "micro dose" of altered state breathwork.

Why would one want to practice altered state breathwork?

You need to have your own answer to this question. Some people believe that it is a path to spiritual enlightenment. Others practice it simply because it feels good. The one thing that I recommend that you do before practicing any form of altered state breathwork is decide on your own "why?"

For me, experiencing an altered state is a powerful disrupter to get me out of my usual way of thinking. It allows me to experience life through a different lens for a moment, and this can be very useful in times of distress, times when I need to make a big life decision, or times when I find myself living in a "funk," a rut, or malaise.

Altered State Defined

So, what is an altered state? It is a state of thinking and feeling that is outside of the norm. Right now, as you are reading this, I assume that you are in a normal state. Your thinking/problem-solving brain is functioning in the same basic way that it does all throughout your day. You have things in the back of your mind, little processes and thoughts that you might not even be aware of, things that affect your mood and state of being. What we do in altered-state breathing is disrupt that process; we restart your consciousness for a moment to provide you with a new way of seeing things.

What to Expect

Many people describe altered state breathwork as psychedelic. I am not going to argue with that definition; however, don't expect to be on a six-hour mushroom trip. The experience will dissipate relatively quickly, so one doesn't have to worry about committing to hours and hours of an altered state.

Experiences will vary. I have listened to what sounded like the voices of a thousand angels singing all around me, enveloping me in a blanket of light. I have also had many experiences where I don't see or hear anything abnormal, but when I open my eyes, I feel a deep sense of connectedness with everyone and everything in the universe. I have also passed out, fallen asleep, or couldn't stop laughing/crying. And there have been plenty of times when nothing much happened.

What you have here in this book allows you to experiment with altered state. If you like it, or if you want to learn deeper or more powerful forms of altered state breathwork, I recommend finding a learned breathworker who can guide you personally through a session. You can book a session with me, or you can find any of the thousands of qualified breathworkers around the world who are trained in an altered state technique.

Best Practices

1. Never do this alone. You should have a partner in this venture to help you through the breathwork and to sit by your side during your altered state experience. You will likely be unable to keep track of time or think about the instructions. Having

a trusted friend to guide you will keep you going and give you a sense of security. This person should also be interested in doing the techniques. **Don't ask someone who is unfamiliar with what you are doing.**

2. Before lying down for your first session, set an intention. Think about the problem you are facing, the feeling that you can't define, the mood that you are stuck in. Decide to dedicate this session to that one thing. Be open to anything that comes, but set the intention to address whatever the thing is that is affecting you in your daily life.

3. Reduce distractions and never do this on a deadline. Prepare to give yourself plenty of time after the breathwork to experience and digest what follows.

4. Never use strobe lights or flashing lights. In fact, low lights are best.

5. Never be in water or in any situation where passing out would cause injury or death.

The "Micro Dose" Altered State Protocol

1. Lie down and become comfortable. Relax your body, and observe your breath.

2. Begin breathing deeply through your nose. Nothing forceful, just deep breaths in and relaxed breaths out through your nose. There should be no pause between breaths, and every exhale should be relaxed.

3. Continue deep breathing through the nose for five minutes.

4. After five minutes of deep nasal breathing, clench the muscles of your pelvic floor (your sexual organs and your anus) while taking one last deep nasal breath fully in.

5. Hold your breath with a full lung for 10 seconds while still clenching your pelvic floor. Apply a light flex to your abdomen.

6. After 10 seconds, exhale and return to normal breathing. Be open to any experience that you have, and take some time to meditate or simply relax.

If you liked that, and you want to see how deep the rabbit hole goes, there are many altered state techniques out there to try. In this written form, the above protocol is all that I am comfortable sharing. Deep altered state breathwork should always be done under the supervision of a trained breathworker who is familiar with altered state breathwork, preferably one who has led others in these kinds of experiences before.

Chapter 29.

Building Your Personal Breathwork Practice

While your breathwork practice should be your own, I recommend at least one or two sessions per day. Here are some things to consider as you create your schedule:

1. **Ideally, breathwork is done on an empty stomach**. You don't have to be hungry, but you don't want to worry about the food in your stomach while focusing on your breathing. In addition to being uncomfortable, the pH changes caused by digestion can affect your results.

2. **Be realistic**. Don't plan to practice a specific amount of breathwork per day if you don't really think you can do it. Remember that it only counts if you actually do it. So, set yourself up for success.

3. **Make posture a priority**. I don't care if you practice breathwork all day every day, if your posture is bad, your results will be suboptimal. There is more to breathing than what is done with your respiratory system. Remember that every time you sit at your desk or look down at your phone.

4. **Morning breathing and pre-bedtime breathing are the best two times of day to begin your practice**. Book-ending your

day with breathwork is generally the best way to get into a consistent practice. You already need to change states, so why not start there? You can always add shorter sessions throughout your day.

Connecting Techniques into a Breathwork Session

All of the techniques discussed in this guide are great when practiced by themselves, but they can also be combined together to create a breathwork session that includes variety and depth. These sessions can go on for long periods of time or just a few minutes. A combined breathing technique session can have a specific goal (i.e. to activate, to relax, to strengthen the diaphragm, etc.) or it can be an exploration of how variations in breathing can create different sensations in the mind and body.

How to Construct a Breathwork Session Out of Multiple Techniques

1. **Before you begin to construct a breathwork session, you should have an idea of what you would like to accomplish.** Do you have a specific goal, or are you just exploring? Perhaps your goal is to work on learning to listen to your "inner voice" (interoception). Great. Now, knowing what you already know, what techniques would you like to use to accomplish this goal?

2. **Decide on an approximate length of time.** In most cases, you will not have unlimited time, so you should think about how long you want your session to last. This will also help you ensure that each technique is being practiced long enough for

its desired effect. If you have to rush through the experience, you'll likely not get much out of it.

3. **Pick techniques to link together and think about the effect that each will have**. What kind of a combination will you create, and how will you link them together in a logical sequence?

4. **Make a plan**. While you may eventually have some sessions where you wing it, planning out sessions before you begin will keep you from drifting and forgetting techniques that you would like to try.

5. **Use music or a metronome for consistent breathing**. A metronome is a great way to ensure that you don't drift as you count during your inhales, exhales, and apneas. Some people say that they use their heartbeat to keep time, but your heart rate may slow or speed up as a result of your breathwork, so it is not a reliable time-keeping device. Another great way of keeping time is to find a musical track with a consistent beat.

6. **Create space in your schedule to fully devote to your session**. Any time we practice breathwork, we are practicing focus and listening (interoception). Don't just go through the motions. Be 100% present with every breath, every count, every moment. If you only have a little bit of spare time, you may want to create a shorter session, or not create a session at all. Remember that you don't have to create breathwork sessions. Individual breathing techniques are still very effective. The key is being devoted and present to your practice.

7. **After your session, take time to reflect**. How did the session go? Was it rushed? Did your techniques clash, or did they fit together perfectly? How do you feel? Did you get the desired

effect? Or do you need to tweak something for your next session? Did you experience changes that you liked? Ask yourself these questions and examine the session. What worked? What needs to be changed? What can you learn?

Sample Activation Breathwork Session | 21 Minutes Duration

Find a seated or lying down position. Close your eyes, and relax your body while keeping a neutral spine.

Self Examination	1 minute	(No change to breathing, just listening)
Four Deep Breaths	30 seconds	(To open up the lungs and begin)
Box Breathing	2 minutes	(To balance the ANS and warm up)
Kapalbhati	2 minutes	(To activate, strengthen breathing muscles, clear sinuses)
Four Deep Breaths	30 seconds	(Relaxes breathing muscles)
Top Triangle	4 minutes	(To activate and to open lungs)
Superventilation	2 minutes	(To activate and to create CO_2 deficit)
Neutral Lung Apnea	90 seconds	(Hypoxic training, ANS Balancing)
Superventilation	2 minutes	(To activate and to create CO_2 deficit)
Neutral Lung Apnea	90 seconds	(Hypoxic training, ANS Balancing)
Top Triangle	4 minutes	(Activation)

Return to normal breathing and observe the changes. Remember that you are an individual. As I stated earlier, even though this combination will be very energizing for most people, since we have so much variation in our species, you might have a different reaction. Ultimately, we have to test sequences in our bodies to know their impact.

Sample Relaxation Breathwork Session | 20 Minutes

Find a seated or lying down position. Close your eyes, and relax your body while keeping a neutral spine. It is especially important to use the nose for all inhales. I recommend using the mouth for all of the exhales because pursing your lips can make lengthening the exhales much easier.

Self Examination	1 minute	(No change to breathing, just listening)
Four Deep Breaths	30 seconds	(To open up the lungs and begin)
Box Breathing	2 minutes	(To balance the ANS and warm up)
Bottom Triangle	4 minutes	(Sends a strong parasympathetic signal)
4,0,8,0 Cadence	3 minutes	(Vagal stimulation, parasympathetic)
Peaceful Apneas	30 seconds	(Allows for complete relaxation)
6,0,10,0 Cadence	3 minutes	
Peaceful Apneas	30 seconds	(Allows for complete relaxation)
10,0,10,0 Cadence	4 minutes	
Peaceful Apneas	30 seconds	(Allows for complete relaxation)
6,0,8,0 Cadence	1 minute	

Return to normal breathing and observe the changes. Remember that you are an individual. Even though this combination will be very relaxing for most people, since we have so much variation in our species, you might have a different reaction. Ultimately, we have to test sequences in our bodies to know their impact.

Sample Athletic Performance Breathwork Session (Hypoxic Training Focus) | Approximately 25 Minutes

Find a seated or lying down position. Close your eyes, and relax your body while keeping a neutral spine. I recommend using the nose for all inhales and the mouth for all exhales.

NOTE: On the post-superventilation apneas, one should never strain to keep from breathing. If you must breathe, simply take a small sip of air, then go back into the remainder of the apnea.

Self Examination	1 minute	(No change to breathing, just listening)
Four Deep Breaths	30 seconds	(To open up the lungs and begin)
Box Breathing	2 minutes	(To balance the ANS and warm up)
Kapalbhati	2 minutes	(To activate, strengthen breathing muscles, clear sinuses)
Full-Lung Apnea	1 minute	
Kapalbhati	2 minutes	(To activate, strengthen breathing muscles, clear sinuses)
Full-Lung Apnea	1 minute	
Superventilation	2 minutes	(To activate and to create CO2 deficit)
Neutral Lung Apnea	90 seconds	(Hypoxic training, ANS Balancing)
Superventilation	2 minutes	(To activate and to create CO2 deficit)
Neutral Lung Apnea	90 seconds	(Hypoxic training, ANS Balancing)
Superventilation	2 minutes	(To activate and to create CO2 deficit)
Neutral Lung Apnea	2 minutes	(Hypoxic training, ANS Balancing)
Inhale, Full-lung Apnea	30 seconds	(Activating)
Four Deep Breaths	30 seconds	(To open up the lungs)
Box Breathing	2 minutes	(To balance the ANS)
4,7,8,0 Breathing	8 repetitions	(Create state of "Stay and Play")

Can I go longer? Sure! All of these are just examples of configurations that have worked for me in the past. When I lead groups, I normally go for around 45 minutes. These classes are usually meant to leave the practitioners with a sense of relaxed wellbeing by the end, but I also try to include various techniques that will improve their health and wellbeing.

Example General Wellbeing Breathwork Sequence

Find a seated or lying down position. Close your eyes, and relax your body while keeping a neutral spine. I recommend using the nose for all inhales and the mouth for all exhales.

Self Examination	1 minute	(No change to breathing, just listening)
Four Deep Breaths	30 seconds	(To open up the lungs and begin)
Box Breathing	2 minutes	(To balance the ANS and warm up)
Kapalbhati	2 minutes	(To activate, strengthen breathing muscles, clear sinuses)
Four Deep Breaths	30 seconds	(Relaxes breathing muscles)
Top Triangle	4 minutes	(To activate and to open lungs)
Superventilation	2 minutes	(To activate and to create CO_2 deficit)
Neutral Lung Apnea	90 seconds	(Hypoxic training, ANS Balancing)
Superventilation	2 minutes	(To activate and to create CO_2 deficit)
Neutral Lung Apnea	90 seconds	(Hypoxic training, ANS Balancing)
Superventilation	2 minutes	(To activate and to create CO_2 deficit)
Neutral Lung Apnea	90 seconds	(Hypoxic training, ANS Balancing)
Full Lung Apnea	30 seconds	(Extend the inner silence)
4,7,8,0 Cadence	2 minutes	(Create a "Stay and Play" state)
4,0,8,0 Cadence	3 minutes	(Vagal stimulation, parasympathetic)
Peaceful Apneas	30 seconds	(Allows for complete relaxation)

6,0,10,0 Cadence	3 minutes	
Peaceful Apneas	30 seconds	(Allows for complete relaxation)
10,0,10,0 Cadence	4 minutes	
Peaceful Apneas	30 seconds	(Allows for complete relaxation)
6,0,8,0 Cadence	2 minute	
6,0,10,0 Cadence	2 minutes	(Add an audible hiss to the exhale)

Example Breathwork Session to Induce a Parasympathetic State and Improve Diaphragm Neuromuscular Control

Find a seated or lying down position. Close your eyes, and relax your body while keeping a neutral spine. I recommend using the nose for all inhales and the mouth for all exhales.

The challenge in this session is to perfectly measure your inhales and exhales, to become in tune with your breathing so much so that with each change in cadence, you do not need to rethink your next breath. Each breath should be fluid and relaxed.

Self Examination	1 minute	(No change to breathing, just listening)
Ocean Breathing	10 slow breaths	
5,0,5,0 Cadence	2 minutes	
6,0,6,0 Cadence	2 minutes	
7,0,7,0 Cadence	2 minutes	
8,0,8,0 Cadence	2 minutes	
9,0,9,0 Cadence	2 minutes	
10,0,10,0 Cadence	2 minutes	
Peaceful Apneas	30 seconds	

Breathing Sessions to Strengthen
Breathing Muscles

These sessions can be done in a seated position or lying down. These sessions can be quite intense at first, so don't feel bad if you don't make it all the way through. If your diaphragm is sore after practicing, wait a few days before trying again, and when you do try again, just remember to try to reduce your intensity a little.

Warrior Lung (Level 1)

Reverse Straw (short)	30 seconds
Full Lung Apnea	30 seconds
Two deep resetting breaths	
Reverse Straw (short)	30 seconds
Full Lung Apnea	30 seconds
Reverse Straw (short)	30 seconds
Full Lung Apnea	30 seconds
Kapalbhati (slow)	1 minute
Full Lung Apnea	30 seconds
Kapalbhati (moderate pace)	1 minute
Full Lung Apnea	30 seconds
Kapalbhati (fast)	1 minute
6 Deep breaths (In nose, out mouth)	
Kapalbhati (any speed)	1 minute
Reverse Straw (longest possible)	1 minute
Neutral Lung Apnea	30 seconds
Reverse Straw (longest possible)	1 minute
Neutral Lung Apnea	30 Seconds
Box Breathing	2 minutes

Warrior Lung (Level 2)

Ocean Breathing	1 minute
Kapalbhati (any speed)	1 minute
Full Lung Apnea	30 seconds
Kapalbhati (any speed)	2 minutes
Full Lung Apnea	30 seconds
Kapalbhati (any speed)	1 minute
Full Lung Apnea	30 seconds
Reverse Straw (short straws)	1 minute
Reverse Straw (long straws)	1 minute
Reverse Straw (longest possible)	1 minute
Neutral Lung Apnea	1 minute
Ocean Breathing	1 minute
Reverse Straw (short straws)	1 minute
Reverse Straw (long straws)	1 minute
Reverse Straw (longest possible)	1 minute
Neutral Lung Apnea	1 minute
Ocean Breathing	1 minute
Box Breathing	2 minutes

Kasper van der Meulen's "Focus Reset Breathing"

Kasper van der Meulen has a talent for creating incredibly simple and short sessions that are easy to add whenever you need them. He shared one with me that he created, based on Box Breathing. He takes the box form and lengthens the apneas. The effect is a quick and easy session to reset your ANS for focus.

Balanced Breathing (4,0,4,0)	4 breaths
Box Breathing (4,4,4,4)	4 repetitions

Extended Box (4,8,4,8)   4 repetitions

Suggestions for Your Daily Practice |
A Few Simple Plans

I encourage you to think about what you want to accomplish with your daily practice. Are you looking to break the dopamine feedback loop? Are you looking for a competitive edge in sports? Maybe you are looking for a way to maintain focus or meditate more easily. Whatever you goal, think about how you can use your breath to accomplish these goals. Your practice is your own. You get to decide what your practice will look like. However, I have provided a few daily plans to get you started below. Please do not look at them as prescriptions; they are simply starting points for the practice that you will create for yourself. You may also notice that I do not include any of the mixed sessions that are described in the first part of this chapter. This is because these plans are meant to be simple so that people will follow them daily. Maybe you are ready to jump into regular sessions like those described above. That is great! Maybe you're not. That is fine! The plans described below should not take much time out of your day, and they can serve as great templates to build your eventual personal daily routine from.

The Daily Dopamine Loop Escape Plan

Morning Session

Ocean Breathing   1 minute

Box Breathing   2 minutes

Any Superventilation technique

you like for three rounds Meditation   5 minutes

Midday Session

4,7,8,0 Breathing   8 rounds

Or

Box Breathing   2 minutes

Afternoon (at least 2 hours after a meal – only if needed)

Wim Hof Method Technique   3 rounds

Before Bed

4,0,8,0 Cadence   3- 5 minutes (Use Ocean Breathing Technique)

As you grow in your practice, add more techniques as you wish. But just start with this for the first few weeks.

Athletic Performance Plan

Morning

Perform CO_2 Tolerance Exhale Test

Top Triangle   5 minutes (Growing the box as is comfortable)

Extreme Hypoxia SV Technique   3 rounds

Midday

Bottom Triangle   10 minutes (Growing the box as is comfortable)

Pre-Workout

Top Triangle   10 minutes (Growing the box, pushing comfort a little)

Intra-Workout

See Chapter 22 for training ideas

Post-Workout

4,0,8,0 Breathing   5 minutes (Use 90/90 Position)

Before Bed

4,0,8,0 Cadence   3- 5 minutes (Use Ocean Breathing Technique)

As you grow in your practice, add more techniques as you wish. But just start with this for the first few weeks.

Plan for Times of Anxiety

Morning

Wim Hof Method Technique	3 rounds
Meditation	5 minutes

Mid- Morning

4,7,8,0 Cadence (Cadence of Happiness)   8 rounds

Midday

4,7,8,0 Cadence (Cadence of Happiness)   8 rounds

Afternoon (at least 2 hours after a meal – only if needed)

Wim Hof Method Technique   3 rounds

Mid-Afternoon

4,7,8,0 Cadence (Cadence of Happiness)   8 rounds

Before Bed

4,0,8,0 Cadence   3- 5 minutes (Use Ocean Breathing Technique)

As you grow in your practice, add more techniques as you wish. But just start with this for the first few weeks.

Do you have a goal? How will you plan your breathwork routine to accommodate your goal(s)? And don't forget, breathwork isn't simply something that we do a specific time of the day. We are always breathing, always training, always informing our nervous system of our state. Every breath counts.

Creating Your Own Breathing Technique

Remember that while there are countless breathing techniques out there, none of this is magic. Breathwork practitioners who have come before you were simply using what they learned from their teachers and their own experiences to produce the breathing techniques that we know today. They didn't ask for permission, nor did they graduate from a university of breathwork. They listened to their inner voice and experimented. Their laboratory? Their own bodies and minds. Breathwork is your birthright. You don't have to wait for a guru. Let your interoception guide you.

Suggestions for Creating Your Own Breathwork Protocol

1. **Experiment over time**. Remember that nothing happens in a vacuum. As you experiment with breathing techniques, always be aware of your internal state as it exists within your current context. Remember that everything that is going on in your life is affecting the way you feel. This means that you should experiment over time, and be observant.

2. **Be honest with your results**. Ask yourself, "What do I expect?" After reading about the elements of breathing, you should have a good idea of how to affect your state using your breath. When you construct your own breathing protocol, you will likely have an intended effect in mind. When you experiment, does the result match the intended effect? Be

honest with yourself, and be willing to make adjustments or even throw away ideas that are not working for you.

3. **Document your creations**. Try to describe your breathing protocol using the four corners of breath notation that we learned earlier in this guide. This is not for the sake of making you think "inside the box"; instead, think of breathwork notation as the language with which you will share your technique with the world. You can add elements such as "pursed lips" or "using a clicking sound." Countless people around the world are practicing breathing protocols that were created thousands of years ago, and this would not be possible if they didn't take the time to document what they created.

4. **Journal**. If you are serious about creating your own protocols, you will need to be able to remember subtle changes that occur, sometimes instantly and sometimes over time. Journaling is a way to document your research.

When you feel that you have created something useful, share it! This is important for two reasons. For one, we want to share good things with others. But, secondly, you will want to see if your new protocol is something that works for others. Remember that we are all very different. It could be the case that you have created a protocol that will help millions of people. But it may also be that your protocol is something very personalized for you. Both are great. Your protocol doesn't have to be good for the masses to have value to you, though it is useful to test it out with multiple people and find out for sure.

How far can I take this?

At this point you are equipped with the fundamental elements of breathwork. You should understand how the techniques described thus far work to influence the body and mind. One of the questions I remember asking myself early on was this: can I just go make up my own breathing technique, armed with the knowledge of what each part of the breathing process will produce? The answer is yes. That sentence should be: There is no magic code; there are only the principles behind each part of your breathing technique, combined with your sense of interoception and your ability to focus. If you can master these things, you can create your own breathing techniques, or combinations of various techniques, and find your own way. Maybe someday you will write your own book based on your discoveries. I would love to read it.

For workshops, retreats, speaking engagements, online videos, and much more, please visit: www.jessecoomer.com

Use the code below for discounts off of most events and products found on www.jessecoomer.com

Special Code: 8XO0Fq1C3CCo2

References

» Barnai, M., Laki, I., Gyurkovits, K., Angyan, L., & Horvath Gyöngyi. (2005). Relationship between breath-hold time and physical performance in patients with cystic fibrosis. *European Journal of Applied Physiology, 95*(2-3), 172–178. https://doi.org/10.1007/s00421-005-1350-3

» Gerritsen, R., & Band, G. (2018). Breath of Life: The Respiratory Vagal Stimulation Model of Contemplative Activity. *Frontiers in human neuroscience, 12*, 397. https://doi.org/10.3389/fnhum.2018.00397

» Herrero, J. L., Khuvis, S., Yeagle, E., Cerf, M., & Mehta, A. D. (2018). Breathing above the brain stem: volitional control and attentional modulation in humans. *Journal of Neurophysiology, 119*(1), 145–159. https://doi.org/10.1152/jn.00551.2017

» Lundberg J. O. (2008). Nitric oxide and the paranasal sinuses. *Anatomical record (Hoboken, N.J. : 2007), 291*(11), 1479–1484. https://doi.org/10.1002/ar.20782

» Melnychuk, M. C., Dockree, P. M., O'Connell, R. G., Murphy, P. R., Balsters, J. H., & Robertson, I. H. (2018). Coupling of respiration and attention via the locus coeruleus: Effects of meditation and pranayama. *Psychophysiology, 55*(9), 1. https://doi-org.dbprox.vinu.edu/10.1111/psyp.13091

» Nishino, T. (2009). Pathophysiology of dyspnea evaluated by breath-holding test: studies of furosemide treatment. *Respiratory Physiology & Neurobiology, 167*(1), 20–25. https://doi.org/10.1016/j.resp.2008.11.007

» Ruth, Alan. (2015) The Health Benefits of Nose Breathing. *Nursing in General Practice.* http://hdl.handle.net/10147/559021

» Semenza, G. L., & Wang, G. L. (1992). A nuclear factor induced by hypoxia via de novo protein synthesis binds to the human erythropoietin gene enhancer at a site required for transcriptional activation. *Molecular and Cellular Biology, 12*(12), 5447–54.

» Stanley, N. N., Cunningham, E. L., Altose, M. D., Kelsen, S. G., Levinson, R. S., & Cherniack, N. S. (1975). Evaluation of breath holding in hypercapnia as a simple clinical test of respiratory chemosensitivity. *Thorax, 30*(3), 337–43.

» Travis, F., Blasdell, K., Liptak, R., Zisman, S., Daley, K., & Douillard, J. (1996). Invincible Athletics program: aerobic exercise and performance without strain. *The International journal of neuroscience, 85*(3-4), 301–308. https://doi.org/10.3109/00207459608986691

» Wang, S. Z., Li, S., Xu, X. Y., Lin, G. P., Shao, L., Zhao, Y., & Wang, T. H. (2010). Effect of Slow Abdominal Breathing Combined With Biofeedback on Blood Pressure and Heart Rate Variability in Prehypertension. *Journal of alternative and complementary medicine (New York, N.Y.), 16*(10), 1039–1045. https://doi.org/10.1089/acm.2009.0577

Printed in Great Britain
by Amazon

31862588R00118